FIT AT ANY AGE

IT'S NEVER TOO LATE

SUSAN NIEBERGALL

have helped me realize that menopause is
an excuse for weight gain. Women over
CAN lose and build muscle

-Kathy, Indianapolis, Indiana

You have inspired me to lift
heavy things at my age! (58
ears YOUNG)

-Traci, Nashville, Ten...

Definitely my favorite saying I've learned from you i

Nutrition is the driver, and exercise is the passenger.
I use this saying all the time!

As well as it's never too late and you're never too old

Beth Thomaston, Mai...

sistency. That is what I
ned. I always gave up.
is time I have not. The weigh
s not coming off as quickly a
would like but I am being

I learned that physical and men
strength can happen at any age!

-Chrissy, Anna...

Here are the main thin
I learned from you:

Form/technique over eg

Consistency is key

Age is literally a social
construct; it is just a num

-Janani, Toro...

Susan keeps it real! It's not about
perfection, but consistency.

Life happe
right bac

hat I have learned from my a
s. Susan ...to keep going even when the s
t moved and to implement rest days.

Love you Ms. s.

When I started my
bulk, I listened to you
advice on the podcas
with Jordan. I learne
a lot from that.

-Jesper, Denma...

At 52, your advice has changed my views on everything.

No gimmicks, just solid, stable, doable advice

--Stephanie, El Paso, Texas

You've taught me so much, but the best things: It's never too late to s[t]
Now is the best time to start no ma[tter]
what.

Second, learn from the best. Soak up [w]hat you can from them an then teach [ot]hers what you've learned. Teach for [...] teach with love and grace and [...] And teach without [...] in return.

[...]
[n]utrition even after many years of not [s]ucceeding with one or both.

[...]ing your strength gains and sheer [b]ass-ness, even though you're olde[r] [n]o offense at all, I'm 54) and a REAL [p]erson, not a fitness competitor, influe[...] whatever, has made me believe it's no[t] only possible, but very attainable.

-Serena, Pennsyl[vania]

Seeing Susan workout has helped and inspired me as a[n] 'older lady', lifting weights isn't just for the young

-Luci[e]

Something I have learned from you, I have reduced cardio, and increased protein. I always though I needed to do lots of cardio.
-Pat, Ireland

I have changed my approach to working because of you.

I have changed my frequency and inte[nsity] for each workout a[nd] I embrace rest da[ys]

-Mary, St. Jo[hn]

Susan,
You bring tough love and honor to the "calorie [...] equation. You've comforted us who thought we h[ad] thyroid problems (nope, just big jaw problems) ... [o]ur shared experience. Thank y[ou ...] [em]pathy along wit[h ...]

The advice in this book has been carefully considered and checked by the author.
It should not, however, be regarded as a substitute for medical advice.
I recommend talking to your doctor before starting any new exercise routine.

DEDICATION

This book is dedicated to my husband Tim and my son Mike (and even Snowball and the late Rascal) who have put up with me all of these years and who have supported this project as well as my fitness and business journeys every step of the way.

CONTENTS

FORWARD

In January of 2016 I was living in Tel Aviv, Israel.

25 years old, renting an apartment overlooking the Mediterranean Sea, and coaching people online from all over the world…I didn't think my life could get any better.

Then I met Susan Niebergall. And my life quickly got better than I ever could have imagined.

We "met" over the internet when Susan e-mailed me asking for online coaching.

At 54 years old, she wanted to get strong. Very strong. Stronger than she'd ever been before. She told me she wanted to get into the sport of Powerlifting. Which, candidly, there weren't many women doing period. Never mind a 54 year old women.

But that's what separated Susan from anyone I'd ever met. And, to this day, it's still what separates Susan from anyone I know.

She didn't care about her age. She didn't use it as an excuse or justification to stop trying. If anything, it became a source of motivation. An opportunity to prove to her and everyone around her that you can get stronger, leaner and in the best shape of your life at any age. That it, truly, is never too late.

And that's exactly what she's done.

When we first started working together, Susan told me she wanted to be able to do a chin-up. A real, unassisted chin-up. She had never been able to do one before but was determined to make it happen.

Several months later, Susan sent me a video of her doing a real, unassisted chin-up. Not long after that, she was doing 3 unassisted chin-ups. Soon thereafter, 5 in a row. Nowadays, at 60 years young, Susan is doing weighted chin-ups with 45 pounds strapped around her waist.

When we first started working together, Susan told me she wanted to be able to Deadlift 200lbs. She wasn't sure if it was going to be possible but she sure as hell would give it her best shot.

On April 11, 2016 (four months after we began), Susan sent me a video of her Deadlifting 245lbs.

I don't share these stories of Susan to impress you. My purpose isn't to convince you of how amazing Susan is or how remarkable all of her accomplishments are.

The reason I'm sharing these stories with you is because, as you'll read in this book, Susan is a normal person just like you and me. She has overcome extraordinary battles to get to where she is today. And she has fought tooth and nail to achieve each and every one of her goals.

It hasn't been easy for Susan. Just as I'm sure it hasn't been easy for you.

But just because it hasn't been easy doesn't mean it's not possible. And it definitely doesn't mean you should give up.

In the following pages you're going to learn more about Susan. She's going to let you in on the good and the bad. She's going to show you where she's succeeded and where she's failed. She's going to walk you through her journey from then until now.

And in each and every one of these pages, you're going to learn more about yourself. You're going to find strength, hope and inspiration to become the best version of yourself. And just as Susan changed my life for the better, so too she'll change yours.

- Jordan Syatt

INTRODUCTION
FIT AT ANY AGE

I felt pure despair. I couldn't understand how I had gained weight again, especially when I thought I was doing everything right. It was the kind of despair where you just want to say, "screw it," and eat all the things. Because it really didn't matter anyway. It seemed as if every attempt I made to lose some weight and lean out didn't work. I was tired of the infamous Yo-Yo diet, where I would lose some weight, regain some, lose again, gain again over and over and over. I wanted out.

I was looking for something to blame it on. Anything. Anything but myself.

I had reached the infamous stage of middle age where your body decides to take over and it does whatever it wants to do, regardless of how you try to direct it. That's what happens, right? Our metabolism slows way down, and that's the primary culprit for our middle-aged belly.

Or, that's what I thought. Or maybe, more accurately said, that's what I wanted to believe, because blaming my current state on something else was way easier than taking responsibility.

Whenever I looked at myself in my bathroom mirror, I always thought, how did this happen to me?

I had pretty much given up and resigned myself to the fact that my current state was as good as it was going to get. My body was being stubborn. No matter what I did, it wouldn't budge.

The level of stubbornness I felt?

Imagine taking a dog for a walk. You leave the house with the dog, and the dog gets to the driveway and decides it doesn't want to take another step. Not one more. He just sits there, in all of his stubbornness, not moving at all. And you keep yanking on the leash, but this dog is a big dog, and he ain't going anywhere.

He's too big to carry, and he will not move. (Actually, if you have a cat, it's more like the stubbornness that a cat shows, every day, all the time.)

That's kind of how it feels when you hit middle age—like everything has come to a screeching halt, and what used to work doesn't work anymore. In a word, I felt stuck.

Now what do I do?

This feeling had been with me for a long time, but for some reason, one particular day, it all spilled over. My clothes were fitting tighter, I was exhausted from working out, and I felt like no matter how hard I pushed myself I was still going nowhere.

It was exhausting. I had been on a Yo-Yo diet, and I miraculously lost weight for a short period of time, but was never able to keep it off. My weight just kept Yo-Yoing up and down. When I was on the low end, I felt great. I felt successful. I felt like this time, it was going to be different. I was going to finally be able to keep it off. But it never turned out that way.

My journey is not unlike anyone else's, really. Mine is, unfortunately, a pretty common story.

That's exactly why I wanted to share my story with you—because I think you will relate to it. I also want to empower you. I want you to see all of the mistakes I made along the way (and trust me, there were plenty), and ultimately I want you to see how I changed it all, while I was well into my fifties. Most importantly, I want you to learn how you can do it, too.

I am an average person, living an average life that started in a very typical household in the sixties. I grew up to have a family of my own, and struggled with my weight on and off for almost my entire life. And when I say "struggled," I don't mean I was ever morbidly obese. The term used back then was "heavy." I tended to be heavy.

I lived through many different fitness "fads," and admittedly got caught up in most of them. I tried Jenny Craig. I tried running. I tried step classes. I tried Aerobics classes. I even tried those chocolate squares that were supposedly appetite suppressants. Newsflash: they were just chocolate squares. They didn't suppress anything.

I finally found lifting, which (though I didn't know it at the time) changed my life completely.

Eventually.

It wasn't the Eureka moment where the skies opened up and the gods above sang in sweet harmony. Lifting was a journey in and of itself, but boy did it change everything.

"Age is just a number" may sound a little sentimental, but there's truth there. We are limited by our own beliefs. I truly believe that, and that's another reason why I wanted to write this book. I don't want a single middle aged woman (or man) to feel like they can't change how they feel, or how they look.

As we get older, so many things feel like a challenge. We can't eat the same way we used to, we don't seem to be able to move like we used to, our bodies seem to have said enough of it all. It would be easy to sit down like that stubborn dog and say, "Welp, it was a good run," then just let Mother Nature have at it.

However, I'm here to tell you that no matter how big of a mountain it seems to be, no matter how overwhelming it may feel, it is totally possible to make changes. We are used to thinking it has to be all or nothing, but that's not how it is.

You may feel like you have a laundry list of things to change and have no idea where to start. The all or nothing mentality creeps in, and pretty soon, the overwhelm takes over. I like to call this moment "paralysis by analysis." You start to think if you can't completely change everything all at once, why bother changing anything at all?

As an online strength coach, I talk to thousands of women who are struggling to lose weight. They all want to make changes, but they often don't know how, or which changes to make. I didn't know either, so I can relate to the frustration that comes with not knowing where to start, or not knowing what to change to make. I know what it's like to think you are doing everything right, yet not see any results. I suffered like that for years and years, and it has since become my passion to help women to finally figure it out, as I finally did.

This all or nothing mentality comes up more times than I can say in phone consults and even in conversations with my clients and Inner Circle members. We always come back to this: Take Action, and Keep Going.

Specific ways you can do this will be explained in the rest of the book, but for now, just know that any change always starts with taking action.

If you are unhappy with how things are for you in the present, don't keep doing the same thing over and over again, expecting a different result. Make a change. Take action. Sure, it's scary. Sometimes we allow the fear to keep us entrenched where we are, but if we want change, we have to take that first step.

Change, for most people, isn't easy on a good day, but it's even more challenging as you get older. You become stuck in your ways, strangely comfortable in your familiar misery. You are willing to endure your misery more than you are willing to change. You may want to change, but you are not willing to change. There's an important distinction there.

If you are willing to change despite the fear of trying something new, and if you can realize that it's going to be a bumpy road but push forward anyway, you will pop out the other side a stronger and more confident person.

Failure is probably the scariest part, and it is something I think we all need to embrace more in life. If we keep setting ourselves up so we don't fail by not trying new things, or by not getting out of our comfort zone, there we will sit. Making excuses as to why things don't work for us. Continuing to unnecessarily endure unhappiness, as well as, maybe, even depression or anxiety.

The great news here is that we do have choices. We can make changes.

And if there is one thing I want you to get from this book, above all else, it is this:

It's never too late to change anything. It doesn't matter how old you are, or what background you are coming from, or what change you want to make, If you want to change, you can.

I did it, and I can show you how to do it, too.

And I am here to support you, every step of the way.

CHAPTER 1
GROWING UP

I was not an obese child. Not at all. I didn't spend most of my childhood thinking about how I looked, or how I wanted to look. I don't have many early memories of social pressures to be or look a certain way. Things were way different back in the sixties and seventies. We didn't have social media (or even computers, for that matter), so I wasn't bombarded with constant ads running 24/7 on the latest and greatest diet, workout, fashion, etc.

Don't get me wrong, there were cliques in school—the popular crowd versus the outcasts. The desire to belong was always there.

I considered myself a member of both groups. I got along with everyone, and always felt sorry for kids who were shunned by the "cool" kids. Maybe that was an early sign of what I would end up focusing on for the majority of my life.

I was born in Arlington, Virginia. My mom, Betty, was a stay at home mom, which back then was the norm. My dad, Earl, was a practicing attorney, ran a law office, and was a substitute judge. I have one older brother, Earl Jr. who is three years older than me.

I knew my dad helped a lot of people as an attorney, but I had no idea just how many people he helped along the way until much later in life, after his death. My desire to help people started with him.

One of my very first memories is getting our family dog. My dad came home with a small white poodle, and I instantly fell in love with that little bundle in his arms. I'm not sure if he cleared it with my mom first or not, but it was too late by that point. Andy was officially a member of the Shaffer family.

Years later, I found out that Andy was given to my dad by a client. I'm not sure if this person couldn't afford to pay my dad or if the dog was just a gift, but things like that happened often.

There were many, many people who couldn't afford an attorney who my dad helped for free. These people didn't end up with my dad because the court appointed him to defend them; he just chose to help them, on his own. Numerous people throughout the course of my life have come up to me and to tell me what a wonderful man my dad was.

I was always so proud of him. The more I learned about what he did, the more I realized I am definitely my father's daughter. The desire to help people was ingrained in me early on, and is something that still drives everything I do.

My mom stayed at home and kept our house spotless (except the kids' rooms). She shuttled my brother and me to all our music lessons and took charge of our schedules. She also cooked all our meals and packed our lunches for school.

Food was a big deal growing up. I was very well fed, and loved my mother's food—except when I was forced to eat peas. I hated peas, but I loved green beans, so on the rare occasion we would have both, my brother and I worked a deal. I gave him my peas and he gave me his green beans. To this day, peas are not my favorite vegetable on the planet.

Our meals were really well balanced: a meat of some kind, a vegetable, and a starch. Pretty basic stuff. Casseroles were a big deal too. My mom had more cookbooks and cooking magazines than any human I knew.

While my parents never forced the clean plate rule on us, they highly encouraged it, and they would always tell us to go back and get more. Portions were never an issue. The more the better. They always wanted to make sure we had enough. And when they entertained, there was more food than you could ever imagine. Looking back, I think it was their way of expressing love. With that generation, food wasn't always plentiful, and I believe that played a significant role in how they dealt with food and our family. They wanted to make sure we were never hungry.

My mom was also the Queen of Christmas. Christmas was a BIG deal in our house, and the meal at Christmas was as big of a deal as the selection of gifts. My mom planned everything out on paper, timing out all of the dishes. The spread was enormous. You would always find turkey or ham (or both), green bean casserole (with the crunchy onions on top), mashed potatoes (with who knows how much butter), homemade gravy and some kind of fruit salad. And then there were all of the dessert options. My mom was the consummate baker, so there was never just one dessert option. A pie or cake, and small bite sized options like brownies, magic bars, or lemon bars were always there. I never thought about what I was eating at those special occasion meals, when I was growing up. I just enjoyed myself. That feeling of being present, and enjoying the meal and the company when I was younger disappeared for a period of time in my life and was replaced with anxiety about being able to stay on track for many years. But I eventually re-learned that skill, and came back full circle to enjoying those special times without any shame or guilt.

Whenever we had people visiting for Christmas, my mom always had a gift for them to open. She never wanted anyone to feel left out. The gift may not have been that big of a deal, but Mom wanted to make sure everyone felt included. I noticed how she made a difference very early on, and always loved it. It became ingrained in me as I grew up. To this day, the desire to make sure people feel included is strong in me. I don't want anyone to ever feel left out of anything.

We were a pretty typical family of four. My parents were very active in our lives as kids, and even as we became adults. They encouraged us to try whatever activities we wanted, and supported us by attending games, recitals, concerts, you name it, they never missed a thing. I dabbled in things like little league softball and swimming, and my parents were always supportive and always in attendance. This is something I have tried to emulate for my own son.

My brother and I both loved sports as kids. We are still both huge DC sports fans. As we were growing up, our dad took us to all kinds of DC sporting events. We had season tickets to the Washington Redskins for most of my life, and often attended Washington Senators baseball games. My brother had many of his birthday parties at RFK stadium, where we all had hotdogs, sodas, and birthday cake, and watched the Senators (most likely) lose. The highlight of my brother's day (and his life, up to that point) was to see his name up on the big screen as one of the birthday celebrants in attendance that day.

I was a well-versed sports fan, but the ironic part is that I wasn't athletic at all. My first exposure to organized sports was Little League Softball when I was in elementary school. All my friends played, and my coach was a friend of my parents, so I gave it a shot.

Our team was the Ginos Giants (Ginos was a fast food restaurant back in the day that tried to give McDonald's some competition. They sponsored our team. Some viewed the name as being only a few steps up from Chico's Bail Bonds from The Bad News Bears.

Our team had an A team and a B team. The A team was made up of all of the best players. They knew what they were doing. Very athletic, and very strong. The B team was considered a training team. I was on the B team. I played catcher.

I could catch the ball from the pitcher, no problem, but I couldn't hit. I'm not sure if I ever got a hit in a game. Softball was not going to be my sport, that had become obvious, but I did enjoy the camaraderie of my teammates.

Because I was well versed in the rules of most sports, most people assumed I was an athlete. They were always surprised to hear I wasn't. I felt like I didn't possess the "sports gene" that others seemed to have. I desperately wanted to be an athlete, but it never really materialized for me.

I did have a brief stint on the junior high school Swim Team—because a bunch of friends were on it. I honestly think, looking back, that I was just desperately trying to fit in with the athlete persona I so desperately wanted to have. Sports seemed to be "the thing" that everyone was doing, so I kept trying to do it, too.

I was probably one of, if not, the slowest swimmer on the team, so I didn't have many opportunities to swim in a meet. I think I swam in one maybe two events, and I was always the third swimmer from the team (AKA, the slowest). I thought sports could be my "thing".

I was wrong.

Music ended up being where I fit in. I started playing the flute in fifth grade and never looked back

Much to my parents' delight, I followed right behind my brother Earl and ended up at James Madison University, studying music education. My parents were beyond happy that both my brother and I were studying to become band directors while attending the same University.

I met my future husband at JMU, as well. Tim shared a house with my brother. To say that my family is a JMU family is an understatement.

Here's the roster:
Susan
Tim (husband)
Earl (brother)
Ellen (sister-in-law)

And now we can add our son, Mike to the list, who just graduated from JMU majoring in Music Industry.

I got my first teaching gig right after graduation at the age of twenty-two. The seniors in my band that year weren't that much younger than I was.

I went on to teach high school and elementary band for eight years. As a high school band director, you tend to have the same students for four years, and you really get a chance to know those kids and their families—the good, the bad, and the ugly. I found myself counseling kids who had rough home situations, or who were struggling to get along with teachers (or even their parents). It was then that I decided to pursue a master's degree in School Counseling. I knew that was what I wanted to do.

I spent my entire counseling career at the same school: Kilmer Middle School in Vienna, Virginia. I went through at least seven principals, a lot of assistant principals (too many to remember), six counseling directors, and thousands and thousands of kids.

I jokingly say that most of my days as a Middle School Counselor were dealing with middle school girls, but it's actually the truth. Middle school girls are a trip. They can be the sweetest and meanest people on this earth. They frequented my office quite a bit because they were in a fight with their best friend, and the rumor mills were swirling. "Everyone" knew. If you are familiar at all with middle school girls, you know that rumors and gossip are basically a state of emergency. They were not going to be able to function, much less pay attention in class, until the issue was resolved.

They are the most interesting, most challenging, and most exhausting group of kids to work with, and I say that with all the love in the world for them.

Through all of my years as a teacher and school counselor, I was doing what I loved to do most: help people. I retired from the school system in 2015, after thirty-three years of service in the state of Virginia.

When I was younger and would think of retirement, I thought I would ride off into the sunset, sleep in, drink coffee, leisurely watch the morning TV shows, and maybe even travel somewhere in September, because for the first time in my entire life, I could vacation whenever I wanted.

When you are a student, then a college student, then immediately get your first job as a teacher right after you graduate, you never leave the school calendar. For fifty years, the school calendar was all I knew.

Being in education for as long as I was gave me a clear identity: I was an educator. That's who I was. That's what I was good at. That was all I knew how to do (or so I thought). I was terrified at the prospect of losing my identity when I retired.

What I didn't know was that I had a whole new identity waiting for me, waiting just over the horizon. My life was going to take a turn that I never would have expected. This "just an educator" would soon be building a fitness business and blazing a trail to show all middle aged women it's never too late to change.

My fitness journey spanned decades, and was full of frustration, doubt, and fear. It was full of common mistakes, many of which stemmed from the common misinformation of that time period. But through it all, I found hope and optimism, and was finally able to get the help I needed to change it all.

I was well into my fifties before I found what really worked for me, but my fitness story has its early roots in the 1980s, shortly after I got married.

CHAPTER 2
YO-YO DIETING

Shortly after I got married, in 1985, I started to put on weight. This was not all that surprising. We had gone on a three-week honeymoon to England, Germany, Austria, and Switzerland, back when the dollar was spectacular over there. We were staying in these incredible bed and breakfasts for almost nothing, eating like kings and queens. It was wonderful, but when we came back I had definitely put on a little weight. I didn't mind at first—but then I slowly kept putting on weight over time.

I wasn't paying attention to my diet at all back then. Looking back on that time, I was eating way more calories than my body needed. So, of course, the weight kept coming. I wasn't a step-on-the-scale girl back then (I didn't even own a scale to step on), but I could certainly tell I had put on weight by how my clothes fit (or did not fit, as the case most usually was).

At some point, I decided enough was enough. I wanted to get the weight off. I was tired of my clothes all being snug and uncomfortable. Every time I put on a pair of pants, it was a reminder of the weight I had put on.

I really had no idea what to do, so I checked out all the latest and greatest ways to lose weight. Really, I was looking for the path of least resistance, the easiest way out. That's when I discovered Jenny Craig.

Jenny Craig was fairly new on the scene in the late eighties and early nineties. Jenny Craig was a weight loss nutrition program. You buy their food, eat it, and lose weight. On the surface, it appeared to be exactly what I wanted: super easy and convenient. All the Jenny Craig commercials centered around the amount of food you could eat and still lose weight. It looked absolutely amazing.

I ordered my meals by the week. They were basically "heat and eat," and most only required a microwave. The concept was super exciting for me. It took all of the thinking out of the equation, which is what I thought I wanted. I didn't have to think. At all. Someone told me what to eat to lose weight, and all I had to do was eat what they gave me. Sounded very appealing to me. Just eat. I could do that.

Ultimately, this ended up doing more harm than good.

Jenny Craig assigned me a counselor, whom I met with regularly. My assigned counselor would conduct a check-in, of sorts. How was I feeling? How did I like the food? General questions like that. They also had workshops you could attend that dealt with all kinds of different topics.

I think I went to one. I don't even remember what it was about, but I thought I should go to one, so I did. I don't think I ever went back.

Having someone tell me exactly what to do was what I loved about the program. I truly thought I had found the magic pill, THE way to finally lose weight.

While I was on Jenny Craig, I was hungry. Very hungry. A lot. If I had known then what I know now, that would have been a huge red flag. Hunger while trying to lose weight is normal. Being borderline ravenous most of the time is not.

The food they gave me was on tiny microwavable trays. Everything for your meal was on that tray. The trays reminded me of the part of an airplane meal that is heated. It wasn't much, and it didn't seem as plentiful as their commercials made it seem, but I kept with it.

When all was said and done, I lost close to fifty pounds while on Jenny Craig. I was super pumped about it. *It worked!* People were noticing. I got a ton of compliments on how I looked. People were asking me what I did, and I proudly recommended Jenny Craig. They all said I looked great. I truly thought that this was it!

Happy ending, right? Unfortunately, no. It was just the beginning.

As I mentioned, Jenny Craig told me what to eat, and I ate it. That's why I thought it worked. I was a rule follower, and since I did exactly what they told me to do, I lost weight.

However, I had no idea how many calories I was eating and I was never taught how calories worked. I only knew that I was hungry. Looking back on it with the knowledge I now have, that level of hunger meant I wasn't eating a lot of calories.

All I knew was what they said: this is your dinner, so eat it. This is your lunch, so eat it. Toward the end of my Jenny Craig plan, the amount of food (calories) was reduced for a short period of time. The explanation, I recall, was centered around our bodies "plateauing" to some degree. Eating less food was meant to jumpstart it again.

Once again, if I knew then what I know now, this would have been another red flag.

I was hungry all the time during this phase, and I was miserable. But I stuck through that period, just doing what I was told—and when I was done with Jenny Craig, when I'd lost close to fifty pounds, I remember feeling like I had conquered it, once and for all.

I was super, super happy! People couldn't believe how much weight I had lost in such a short period of time (that should have been yet another red flag).

On the surface, all of this may seem great and motivating, which to some degree it was. I looked completely different, and I felt great. More energy, new clothes, feeling good.

So, if it worked, what's the problem?

The problem with programs like Jenny Craig is that there is no real information about the portion sizes or macros in what you are eating. The bigger issue in general is that you don't learn anything. You don't learn how to survive in the real world. You don't learn about managing your own portion sizes, or about calories at all.

I didn't learn a thing about how to track my food, how much protein would be appropriate for me and my goals, or how to deal with the anxiety of going to a restaurant and not feeling like I was screwing up my progress. There was so much information left on the table, but like I have said, I just didn't know this stuff back then. I fell for all of the marketing; hook, line, and sinker.

I look at it sort of like those weight loss shows where people are losing massive amounts of weight. If those shows had a "Where Are They Now" reunion special, you would most likely see that a majority of the contestants regained most or all of their initial weight, for pretty much the same reason: there was not enough education. To keep weight off, people need to learn more about the mindset behind relationships with food, how to maintain your new weight, and how to manage everyday situations.

One thing I have learned over time is that the faster you lose weight, the less likely you are to be able to keep it off.

So, while I felt like a complete success story at the end of Jenny Craig, ultimately, it didn't work for me because the weight came back. I didn't learn about portion sizes, so I had no idea how much I was eating. I didn't learn how to plan out meals that would meet my goals, how much protein to have, or what kinds of foods I could eat that would keep me feeling satisfied. And I certainly didn't learn how to incorporate any treats, or any of those "fun foods." There was no exit plan. No survival guide on how to move forward in the post-Jenny Craig life.

My weight didn't all come back at once, but that started my big period of Yo-Yo dieting. I started by losing those fifty pounds with Jenny Craig, then, since I didn't know how to maintain it, I watched the weight jump up and down for years afterward.

The weight came back on in different increments. Sometimes it was ten pounds, sometimes it was twenty pounds, sometimes it was losing another ten and then gaining fifteen back. This was over the course of years, not in any short period of time, but the cycle kept going, And the thing was, I never really had a plan for stopping the cycle. I didn't know how. I only did what I knew. I severely restricted calories without knowing how many calories I should actually be eating. All I knew from Jenny Craig was that I was hungry a lot, so being hungry must be the norm when dieting. To follow that logic, I would eat as little as possible, and I would eventually lose weight. I couldn't keep that going (of course), so I would end up increasing portion sizes over time, would overeat, and then I would put more weight back on.

All the while, I was also exercising. Mostly, I was doing things like Jazzercise and group classes at the beginning. Later on, I started to run, and eventually weight train, but I was still spinning my wheels.

There is a ton of shame involved in being a Yo-Yo dieter. I imagine it is similar to the shame a binge eater might feel after bingeing. I wasn't a binge eater, per se, but the feelings of being a failure were the same. It's not something I ever talked about. I didn't want to admit I needed to lose weight—or even worse that I was trying and couldn't do it (consistently). It was a lonely place to be, but when I was on the low end of the Yo-Yo, at my lowest weight, I would get compliments. People thought I had my shit together. And on some level, I thought I did too, and that fueled my fire. But in reality, I didn't have my shit together. I was wandering aimlessly.

When I was at the bottom of a Yo-Yo cycle, I thought, *THIS* time it will be different. *THIS* time *I will keep the weight off.* And for a while, I usually did. But I was so restrictive with how I approached weight loss that it never worked in the long term.

I even went through a SlimFast phase.   Anyone remember that? It was another diet plan that involved a lot of shakes instead of solid food. I thought I was being "good," but this was just another example of me thinking I knew what I was doing. I never gave a second thought to whether or not I could or wanted to eat like I was eating on a long-term basis. I mean, really. A *shake* as the main staple in my diet. What was I thinking?

The honest answer is that I thought these diets were ways to keep calories in control, and to some degree, they were. But I would be ravenous by dinner, and would eat much larger portions than I needed to. I wasn't a binger. I didn't sit and eat food almost uncontrollably. I didn't eat food from a package, or go through my cabinets and eat everything I could get my hands on. That wasn't me.

I was a "healthy" overeater.

Healthy overeaters are always thinking they are doing everything right, because most of the food they eat would be considered "healthy." Consider the SlimFast shake I would have for breakfast, along with some Cherrios. If you were to name a few "healthy" cereals, Cherrios may be at the top of the list. Most everyone thinks Cherrios are at least somewhat healthy, because they don't have any sugar. That's why you see moms giving their older babies and toddlers Cherrios as a healthy snack. Lord knows I had a small Tupperware container filled with Cherrios in the diaper bag while my son, Mike was young. Cherrios were the go-to. It was considered a "good" food.

This "good food" versus "bad food" way of thinking was ultimately my issue. Foods that sounded healthy were what I primarily ate, which, on some level, was at least a step in the right direction. Foods like nuts (I ate A LOT of almonds), healthy fats like peanut butter (and other nut butters), raisins, trail mix, guacamole, smoothies, and anything with the words "whole grain," "multi-grain," or "organic". While there is nothing wrong with any of those foods, they can all be very calorie-dense.

My problem was that I never thought about calories when it came to healthy food. Because, why would I? It was healthy. It was good for me. Cheerios are good for me, so I can eat as many bowls of Cheerios I want, right? Calories never even crossed my mind, nor did the science of how losing weight works.

Marketing plays a huge role in how we think of food. Marketers are really clever at promoting products that are organic, or whole grain, multi-grain, or all-natural.

While there is nothing wrong with any of that from a

nutrient perspective, I would think multigrain pasta was super healthy—so I had enormous portions of it. I'm sure there were health benefits to it, but not in the quantities I was eating.

Granola and trail mix are two other foods that often fall into the all-natural or "healthy" categories. By the time I would finish a big bowl of some type of granola cereal with milk, I would have consumed a super high-calorie breakfast—and would still be hungry an hour and half later.

I would grab multiple handfuls of trail mix (especially the kind with M&Ms in it), thinking this was healthy. It had nuts in it, and nuts are healthy, right? Nuts are a great source of fat, but they also contain a boat-load of calories. I wasn't thinking about that. All I thought about was how cool it was that the healthy trail mix had M&Ms in it and it was *still* considered healthy! Win-win, in my book.

But when all was said and done, multiple handfuls of trail mix throughout the day added anywhere from three to six hundred calories to my diet. It wasn't a meal. It was a snack—most of the time, it was a mindless snack.

Again, I was just spinning my nutrition wheels.

Through the course of the Yo-Yo cycles, I kept thinking to myself that the only way I could get rid of the weight was to exercise more. I was eating healthily, so the problem must be my exercise. I would go to more classes, add more training, add more running. *More* was the answer, and in addition to that, severely restricting food intake. I thought I had the perfect scenario. More exercising, less food. What could possibly go wrong?

I continued to restrict food. Actually, I hardly ate anything, so of course the weight came off—but then, of course, the weight would come right back because I couldn't stick to it. I didn't have a plan. I was just winging it. I was going by what I thought I knew, but I wasn't thinking long-term. I was thinking short-term.

This short term mindset is very common. *If I just lose the weight quickly, I can figure out how to maintain it later,* I thought. *I'll be able to figure that out when I get there, but I just need to get this weight off now.*

The amount of times I hear clients say this to me now is astounding, but I totally get it, because I thought the exact same thing. I even remember thinking, *I'll just go through a few days of not eating much at all, and I will drop some weight that way. And then I'll learn how to maintain it.*

You know how, when you have to do something or face something you don't want to do, you keep putting it off? You find reasons not to do it. You make every excuse in the book. That was me, with learning how I was going to maintain any weight loss. I didn't want to face it, so I didn't. I would figure it out later. I would make it work when the time comes.

Sounds good at first, but the problem is, it never works that way. That time never comes. We think we have control, that we know everything, but we ultimately don't. If we don't learn what we're doing along the way, if we don't put in the work and instead go for the quickest, shortest, most convenient thing we can do, we aren't going to create a way of life that we can sustain forever.

Makes perfect sense, doesn't it? So why did I not see it

that way? I have no idea, other than I just thought I could do it without a real plan, because the next time would be the time it finally all worked.

And so, that was my big issue, I didn't know how to maintain. I would severely restrict calories, lose weight, and then the weight would come back in various increments. I cycled like this for years and years and years. I kept setting myself up for failure, time and time again, by thinking the same pattern would work when it hadn't in the past. And, of course, it never did.

I remember my college band director once using this phrase: if it stinks, don't just sit there and smell it.

What he was referring to was if us musicians could hear that we were out of tune, we should do something about it. Not continue to play out of tune, but to actually change something so we would be playing in tune. On most instruments, you could move a pipe, a slide, or a joint to change the pitch. So you move the joint, and if you sound better, more in tune, you made the right move. If you sounded worse, you went the wrong way. Instead of pulling out the joint, push it in a little.

Our director's point was to do something to fix the problem. Don't sit there and "smell it". Make a change, because what you were doing wasn't working.

That is ultimately what was going on with me. What I had been doing over and over was still not working, but yet I didn't make any significant changes. As a result, I ended up having two sets of clothes in my closet. One set I called my "fat clothes" and the other set I called my skinny clothes.

This is another common characteristic of a Yo-Yo dieter, having clothes in different sizes. When you Yo-Yo diet and your weight goes up and down, sometimes your clothes would fit and sometimes they wouldn't.

I would never allow myself to get rid of the larger clothes. I was subconsciously thinking that I was going to need them again, because that had been my pattern. I was on the lose/gain/lose/gain train. So I kept two full sets of clothes which included everything: work clothes, casual clothes and even workout clothes.

If you are in a Yo-Yo dieting cycle and you live in a part of the country where seasons change, you have a lot of clothes. Here in Virginia, every season brings something different to the table.

One of the most stressful times for me was when the weather started to cool down and I started having to wear jeans or pants instead of shorts. Jeans always gave me anxiety. After spending months with nothing but shorts on my legs, trying on jeans I hadn't worn in months was terrifying. Lord knows, the emergence of skinny jeans made it even worse.

I literally could feel the anxiety creep in when it was time to see what jeans fit and what jeans didn't. If any of you have ever struggled with this, you know exactly what I'm talking about.

I felt like I was squeezing myself into some small little container. They never seemed to fit right. They may fit through the hips, but not the waist. Or the waist was so super tight that I had to suck everything in just to get the zipper up. Then I let out a monstrous exhale and prayed that the button wouldn't pop open.

It made me feel like crap. It was a constant reminder of how I had failed yet again. I refused to buy a size larger than what my "fat clothes" were. I outright refused. To me, that was the ultimate sign of failure, and I just wasn't going to give in.

So instead, I was going to make myself suffer in jeans that did not fit me. That was my punishment for not being able to sustain my weight, and for not fitting into the skinnier jeans. That was a huge mistake. Huge, huge mistake. I see that now, but at the time, I thought my jeans would be my "motivation" to lose the weight again.

Unfortunately, instead of feeling motivated, I felt defeated. Over and over again.

I would, at some point, try to utilize all the clothes in my closet as "motivation." And every single time I would begin to fit into the "skinny clothes," I would think, "This is it. I will never have to wear the other clothes ever again."

Again, I was wrong.

And while we are talking about women's clothing, it's interesting how different brands of women's clothes fit you very differently. One brand, we could be a size six, the next brand we could be a size eight. One brand, we can be a four, the next brand we are a ten. I would always try to find a brand that I would be a smaller size in. It would give me a temporary feeling of happiness and even a sense of accomplishment to some degree; "I can wear a six!!"

I knew logically what clothing designers were doing

-adjusting their sizes so larger people feel better about themselves by basically wearing a smaller number. If I would normally wear a size fourteen, but could suddenly fit into a size six in a particular brand, I would buy that brand ten out of ten times

Having two sets of clothes played with my mind. When I opened my closet, I saw some clothes that I could wear, but also lots of clothes that I couldn't wear. I didn't know what to get rid of, what to keep, or what clothes to even buy. Every single time I opened my closet, I would see a wall of reminders of my latest failure.

At the time, I was thinking I was playing it smart. Having two sets of clothes kept me prepared. Ready for any situation at any size. But what I wasn't aware of at the time was the toll it was taking on me and how I viewed myself. Those feelings of inadequacy would haunt me for years and years.

I was never considered "obese," but I definitely had weight to lose. If you pay attention to those BMI charts (which are general AT BEST) at your doctor's office, I was in the "overweight" category. Sometimes I made it into the "high normal" range. BMI charts are useful if you have significant weight to lose, but for most people, the body fat number is just another number to chase and become obsessed with, like the number on the scale. The lower the number, the more successful we feel. Wanting to get 20% body fat to 19% body fat isn't going to change your health much, if at all, and it's certainly not going to change your life. But for someone who is obese, it could be a matter of life and death. The numbers and the chart could be a much-needed eye opener for that population.

The other issue I have in general with body fat percentages is that, depending on how you get it evaluated, the numbers themselves may not be all that accurate, anyway. Even some of those super expensive tests are not one hundred percent accurate, so certainly the scales in your house that measure your body fat percentage aren't going to be super accurate, either.

I'm not anti-body-fat-percentage. I just caution you to not get too caught up in any number, whether its body fat percentage or the number on the scale.

When I had to use my "fat clothes," it sent a message to me that I was a failure, yet again. My heart would sink when I would have to put on a larger pair of pants. I was humiliated, frustrated, and angry. I kept a lot of these emotions to myself. Never told anyone—not even my husband. To his credit, he always thought (and still thinks) I looked good. He never thought I was fat. This was all self-driven.

This whole cycle of self-hatred when it came to trying on my old jeans in the fall would continue when it was time to try on my old shorts for spring and summer. I was always trying to squeeze myself into clothes that didn't fit as opposed to getting clothes that did fit properly, and always shaming myself when it didn't work. This was a mind game I was playing with myself, and I see it a lot with clients now. We always think that *this* time, it will be different. *This* time, I will make myself so uncomfortable by wearing clothes that don't fit that it will be a daily reminder that I need to lose weight. So, *this* time, I would severely restrict calories—but unfortunately this time, like every time, I continued right along in the Yo-Yo Cycle: restrict food, lose weight, eat a lot of healthy foods, gain weight, try on the jeans, get mad at myself.

I was getting sick and tired of feeling sick and tired, and I was definitely sick and tired of being on the Yo-Yo cycle. I wanted out, but didn't know how to do it.

Then I joined a gym, and I finally thought I had found *the* answer.

CHAPTER 3
MY GYM RAT DAYS

Back in the eighties and nineties, exercising was very different. Back then, there was a big focus on high-impact aerobic classes. Lots of jumping, pounding, loud upbeat music, and of course, the outfits.

I would be remiss if I didn't mention the outfits.

Picture this: bicycle shorts or leggings with a brightly colored thong leotard over top, that may or may not have included a belt and big, droopy socks known as leg warmers.

And if you had a lot of hair (which many did back then), then you had to complete the look by adding the headband with the big hair sticking out of the top. You can Google "aerobics outfits of the nineties" and get the picture. It's hard to fathom ever dressing like that now, but wow, everyone did back then. Lots of bright colors, and lots of layers. You stuck out if you didn't dress like that.

Now they make Halloween costumes to look just like that. You can dress up for Halloween like an nineties aerobics instructor. It's really funny having lived through it.

I didn't have the complete look by any means, but boy, did I try. I remember putting a thong leotard over bicycle shorts and wondering, *how do people do this?* It was incredibly uncomfortable, and I was a bit self-conscious.

OK, a LOT self-conscious.

Having a leotard up my butt was not the look I was after, and it was a bit too form-fitting for me. I never felt like I had the right shape to pull that look off.

I said, "Screw that," and just wore tights or bicycle shorts with another pair of shorts over top. Yes, you heard right. Tights or bicycle shorts, with regular shorts or running shorts over top. At that time, I thought *just* wearing tights or *just* bicycle shorts was a little too edgy for me. I laugh at that now. Fast forward twenty-five years or so, and you will find me wearing only super short shorts and a sports bra more often than not, when I am at the gym

Oh, how times have changed

But that was the time period when I got started.

My introduction to formal exercise was Jazzercise. Jazzercise was a dance fitness class that combined dance with some strength and resistance training to loud, upbeat music. It was held in a fellowship room at a church, and we had to clear tables and chairs before it started. I don't recall a lot of specifics other than that I felt very awkward and was always looking forward to it being over. In reality, it was way more dance-based than anything else and definitely not in my comfort zone, but I gave it a shot.

I remember always feeling very accomplished when it was over. The people there were very friendly, but the fact that I have so little memory of my time doing it speaks volumes to how I felt back then: it really wasn't for me. It was not something I was going to keep up, and it was not something I looked forward to all that much.

My first experience in a proper gym was taking some high-intensity aerobics classes. The classes were all set to music, loosely choreographed, and were basically set up in four parts:

Warm up
Aerobics
Weights
Cool Down

The instructor would stand in front of the class and wear one of those large microphones that was attached to a head piece. It reminded me of when I had just gotten my braces off and had to wear a headgear at night. Super attractive. It was connected to some sort of power source attached to their waist, that ultimately would keep shorting out.

The warm up got you moving around in time with the music. Nothing too crazy. Lots of grapevine moves and hops and claps, complete with yelling "Woo!"

Then came the aerobics segment, which was the majority of the class. Lots of jumping, kicking, dancing, and sweating, as the music blared through the speakers. Everything was choreographed to the music. I was a music teacher at the time, which was a blessing and a curse in a class like that.

It was a blessing because I could appreciate movements that were on a downbeat and worked with musical phrasing. It made the choreography make sense and easier to remember and execute. The instructors who could stay on beat and learn to call out the moves a few counts before had my utmost respect.

It was a curse because when there was an instructor who did not understand musical phrasing and would therefore start a new sequence in the middle of the chorus, it would drive me crazy. I think it drove others crazy, too, but not for the same reasons.

When an instructor got off beat, the entire class struggled. The class was not in sync. Some people didn't even realize they were out of sync; they just kept doing their thing. But being out of sync made everything more difficult for me. It got us all off our internal rhythm (yes, even you all who claim to not have a musical bone in your body, you have internal rhythm, too).

So, I would be *that* annoying student who would perform the choreography the way the instructor *should* have. I couldn't help it. You musicians out there can understand. Any good musician cannot start a new phrase on count two. It's almost impossible. I will leave that there.

During one class, I was standing toward the back and the instructor got off beat (again). It was like torture for me. Like nails on a chalkboard, or the squeaking of styrofoam. It was that bad.

I hopped right back on beat. I was not with the instructor anymore (who was still off beat) and soon, the people next to me went along with me. We had our own little corner of the group on beat, and crushing it. The instructor eventually hopped on board too.

I wasn't doing it to be a rebel, I promise. I just didn't see the purpose of staying off beat, feeling clumsy, and not getting what I could out of the class. Many others felt the same.

When you are on beat or in time with the music, your movements are easier and you can put more energy into what you are doing. If you are clumsily trying to find the beat, it's going to be tougher to bring intensity to your exercise. You will always see the difference in classes that have instructors who are timing the moves to the beat of the music and even the musical phrases, and to those classes whose instructors are not. One class will have way more intensity and energy, while the other will be confused and lackluster. It's an interesting thing to see. Next time you are in a gym and can observe a class that is choreographed, see if you can tell the difference.

The weight-training portion of the class was next. We would grab a pair of dumbbells (usually fairly light) and do a gazillion repetitions, mostly centered on the arms and shoulders. Back then, the music was just background for this section, so staying on/off beat wasn't an issue—but nowadays, there are very popular group classes that choreograph strength training with music. I'm not sure I could handle that.

After the weightlifting portion, we would do a brief round of ab work, cool down, and then we were done. It was an hour-long class, and we all sweat, jumped, danced, and lifted, and then headed to the gym cafe and sat around and chatted. The community piece was huge for me and kept me coming back. That was significant.

Community is an overlooked component of fitness for many people. When you have a group of people who are on a similar path as you, who are sweating with you, who are there cheering you on and pushing you, it can be a game changer. Little did I know that I would be coaching such a group of people thirty years later.

Programs like Crossfit and Orangetheory do the community thing really well. Almost everyone I have ever spoken to about Crossfit speaks highly of the camaraderie and the support from the other members and instructors. That aspect was what kept them coming back. I hear the same thing about Orangetheory. Feeling like you belong and are in a comfortable environment is key to adhering to just about anything. If you hate going, you won't go.

It was the sense of community back in the nineties that got me into the gym four to five times a week. And I loved it. I loved the music, I loved the instructors, I loved the whole gym atmosphere with people working hard. It quickly became my favorite place to be.

While my exercise frequency increased, I may have seen some temporary results in my weight, but because nothing much changed in the nutrition department, things were, more or less, status quo. However, weight aside, I was discovering a newfound love: exercising.

In my gym, the group exercise area was right next to the free weight section, so I could always see what people were doing over there. I was fascinated with everything I saw, and how strong everyone looked. The more I went to the gym, the more I watched the trainers working with their clients, and was envious of the instruction the clients were getting. I kept telling myself I wanted to do that, too. I wanted to learn about weightlifting. Watching people lift weights in the free weight section of the gym looked very different then the weight lifting part of the classes I was taking, and I loved the thought of having a private trainer just for me. I wanted to get stronger.

I spent a lot of time observing the different trainers in the gym and how they interacted with their clients. Being a teacher, I was really in tune with how they were teaching, how they answered their client's questions, and how attentive they were. After a month or so of observing, I decided on the trainer I wanted to work with, and I got the courage to approach him.

David was incredibly kind and was excited to take me on.

Every time I trained with him, I felt stronger. He set me up for success from the beginning, so when I left the gym I felt accomplished. I felt confident, and I couldn't wait for the next session.

I was officially becoming a "gym rat."

The unofficial definition of a gym rat is someone who not only loves working out, but who loves working out in a gym and being in the gym environment.

The gym environment was growing on me. I found my-self excited to go to the gym and to be in that environment. Watching everyone working hard was super motivating to me. Every time I went there, I knew I was doing something good for my body—and that was a huge plus. Now that I had a trainer, I was excited to learn more, and couldn't wait for my next session. If I could have afforded it, I would have worked with a trainer four or five times a week.

This was who I was quickly becoming.

My trainer taught me the basics. I learned how to squat, hinge, press, and pull. We did a combination of free weights and machines. I loved the feeling of getting strong. I worked with David for at least a year, maybe more. He worked with me through my pregnancy—literally just days before I gave birth, I had a training session with him. I remember one of my doctors saying to me afterward, "You need to thank your trainer. You are really strong."

Those words made me feel great, and they sat with me for years.

CHAPTER 4
FINDING EXERCISE AS A NEW MOM: RUNNING

After I gave birth, and as soon as I was given the medical OK to start exercising again, I did. OK, so I may actually have gone a day or two before I was given the go-ahead, but I was chomping at the bit to get back, and I was a little panicked that I was going to lose all the progress I thought I had made.

I started back by walking on a treadmill and slowly increasing the incline and speed. After that, I went back to the weights, but kept things relatively easy for a while. Due to having a newborn, my life had changed dramatically, and I had to change gyms to one that was considerably closer to me. I also had to change my approach to training.

As a new mom, my time had become limited. It was a rare occasion when I had the luxury of going to the gym, taking an hour-long class, or hitting the free weight section on my own. Any new mom will know that even when I did have the time, the energy wasn't always there. The lack of sleep when you have a newborn is outrageous. When I was pregnant, I always heard "sleep when the baby sleeps," but that was about it. No one ever gave any gory details about just how horrible you could feel with such little sleep.

When we first brought Mike home from the hospital, he evidently wasn't too keen on his new digs and didn't want to sleep at all. We had a bassinet right next to the bed so I could easily feed him without having to get out of bed. Sounds great in theory, but maybe not in practice. He cried so much throughout the night that he spent a grand total of one night in our bedroom. I wheeled that bassinet back across the hall to his room, and there he stayed. I figured I could hear him just fine from across the hall (which I definitely could). He never spent a single night in our room thereafter, as a baby or a toddler

On occasion, poor Tim had to take newborn Mike for a drive on the highway late at night, just so he would fall asleep. The humming of the car and the movement helped lull Mike to sleep. The things we did, back then, to get the baby to sleep (and thus allow us to sleep) were all worth it, as I'm sure any parent would agree.

Being a new parent was stressful. There is no manual that comes with a newborn, so new moms are winging it 24/7 and learning every single day. We all hope we aren't messing up our kids for life as we learn how to be a parent, but as we all eventually discover, our kids seem to turn out pretty damn good despite the rookie mistakes we made along the way.

Pretty early on, I was given the gift of a Baby Jogger. The Baby Jogger was going to be my savior: I would be able to exercise and get some of the post-pregnancy weight off, all while taking care of my baby. I was excited to have an option that didn't involve having to pack up the baby and all his stuff, and drive somewhere to workout. I could literally strap him in and go out of my front door.

The Baby Jogger was a gigantic, three-wheeled stroller that was designed with super big wheels to go over any kind of terrain. It had a comfortable seat for a baby/child weighing up to fifty pounds. It also had a basket underneath that could hold anything you would want to take on a jog. It also was semi-easy to fold up and put in the car. Not quite as easy as they demonstrated in the store (isn't that always the case?), but if I could do it fairly easily, I considered that a victory.

For it's time, in 1997-1998, the Baby Jogger was state of the art. The latest and greatest. It was big and bulky, but it moved well, it was easy to push, and the ride was smooth because of the gigantic tires. I am sure the technology behind modern joggers has improved greatly, and they have gotten more compact and efficient. Even basic strollers now are better designed and can be used for jogging, but I didn't have that option back in the day.

I was missing being able to workout regularly, and was anxious to push myself a bit on our walks. I couldn't start using the jogger until Mike could hold his head up (and as a side note, Mike had a HUGE head to hold up. Bless his Niebergall heart. That kid's head was ginormous), so we just took walks for a while. Our first adventures were short walks around the neighborhood. It gave me the chance to get out of the house and move, and it gave Mike the opportunity to be "lulled" into sleep by the motion of the jogger. The jogger wasn't quite as effective as car rides, but for the most part, Mike liked being in it and going for a ride.

As Mike got bigger, and I got used to "driving" the Baby Jogger, we started to pick up the pace. And when I say picking up the pace, let's be clear: it was a slow jog. I was never the best nor fastest runner ever. I was happy just to plod along.

I was excited to start running. I had always heard it was a great form of exercise that burned a boatload of calories. What could be better for a busy new mom? My running "career" was officially born.

On one adventure, when Mike was getting bigger, we set out on our usual course of walking and running. All was going great, until it wasn't.

Any mom will tell you that once the child learns to walk, that's pretty much all they want to do. As a typical toddler might want to do, Mike wanted out of the stroller. He was done with riding, and wanted to get out and move around. He couldn't fully freely walk on his own, yet. Mike was at what I call the "drunken sailor" stage. He staggered around, very unstable, looking like he had taken one too many sips of the "good stuff." Going for a nice, casual walk with a drunken sailor toddler in one hand, and attempting to drive the baby jogger with the other hand, wasn't going to be an easy task.

Luckily, we weren't too far from home at that point, but I was still struggling with Mike staggering around, and trying to control the jogger. Mike refused to get back in the jogger, and I just wanted to get home at this point, so I attempted to carry him, kicking and screaming and driving the jogger. . Needless to say, it was the longest half mile walk of my life.

Despite some challenging moments trying to take Mike with me, I really enjoyed running—though, maybe a better clarification would be that I really enjoyed the idea of running. The freedom of putting on shoes and heading out the door was very appealing. Getting exercise and some fresh air, just by putting on shoes and heading out the door, was liberating. I thought running was the answer to all of my time issues, weight issues, and building muscle issues.

Someone once told me that running was the exercise to change your body shape. I bought into it hook, line, and sinker, only to find out later that it wasn't true at all. I thought running was going to be my ticket to building a strong and lean body, but what wasn't mentioned was the role nutrition plays. Running can affect your appetite and raise the calories you ultimately consume if you aren't on top of it all. Running is hard, and can make you hungry. You think you are burning more calories than you actually are, and it is very easy to overeat after a run. I, like all new moms, wanted to lose the baby weight quickly, and really thought running was my golden ticket for losing the baby weight.

I started by just trying to run. No plan. Just run. See how far I could go. I found out some very important things right away:

1. Running is hard
2. Running with a baby is even harder

3. The first mile is the hardest. It is brutally hard, both physically and mentally
4. Running is hard!

Running was way harder than I thought it would be. I started to gain incredible respect for those who ran races regularly and who could keep up a fast pace. The first mile is the worst. It feels like it takes forever to get into a groove and get your breathing under control. Sometimes I felt like I was going to die and would think, *why in the world do people even like this?*

But as I continued, I grew to tolerate it. I told people I loved it, but I don't think I ever really did. I loved the idea of being a fast runner and being able to better my time, but I don't ever remember thinking, *Damn, I love this, while I was running.*

I entered my first 5K race in D.C. called Race for the Cure, designed to raise money for breast cancer research. In such a gigantic race, I figured I could easily blend in, not be noticed for how slow I was going, and hopefully, not finish last.

My biggest fear was finishing last. Out of tens of thousands of people, finishing dead last would be humiliating. I really didn't want to be *that* person the race crew waited for so they could tear down all of the racing infrastructure. *That* person, who arrives at the post-race festivities just to find out they are over and everyone has gone home.

I think any new runner has visions of those things happening, especially on your first race, but the reality for most everyone is that it won't happen like that, and it didn't for me.

I finished. I was proud. I thought it was hard. The post-race celebration was fun. There was lots of food—bagels, bananas, protein bars, water, and other odds and ends. The music was loud and uplifting, and the crowd was massive and super friendly. I felt like I had been a part of a big, important event. It was fun. I decided right then and there that I wanted to try more races, and maybe even longer distances.

It had to get easier, right? Someone once told me, if you can do a 5K, you can do a 10K, so a 10K was my next stop. I also decided I would actually "train" for it, in some kind of logical progression. There were some new apps appearing that helped you set up a very basic training program. They told you how far to run on what days. There was even an app that would sync your music to a specific number of beats per minute (bpm) based on your running stride. While the app I tried wasn't all that reliable (lots of bugs, etc.), this former music teacher appreciated being able to run in sync with music. For me, it made running easier and way more fun.

It was about this time that I discovered Jeff Galloway, an expert running coach who had written several books on running and talked a lot about his "Run Walk Run" method.

Just the name appealed to me. Jeff was a little older than I was, and had been crushing the running scene for years. I started looking into this concept and found it was a great fit for me.

The premise is that you divide up your run with periods of running and periods of walking the entire way. The walking periods could be for specified time, or for a specified distance. The whole point was to start the intervals out of the gate, and not wait until you felt like you "needed" them (a BIG mistake I made later on).

As I started training for 10Ks, I implemented this technique. It helped me a great deal, especially with the mental piece that was extremely difficult at the beginning. Make no mistake, I was still slow—very slow—but running was becoming a bit more doable.

One thing I started to discover about the running community was that they appeared to put a lot of importance on whether you ran the whole race or not. It was like it was some sort of badge you could proudly wear after a race, and if you didn't run the whole thing, you were somehow "less than." Every time I would engage in a conversation with an experienced runner, almost without fail, the runner would ask me this:

"Did you run the entire race?"

Why no, I did not. Ever. There was a look of, "Oh," and a silence that was deafening. Invariably, I would get a comment back like, "Oh, you'll get there," or something equally as condescending. The issue was, I WAS there. This was where "there" was for me. This was where I liked it. This was where I had the most confidence. But I guess for some of the running community, Run Walk Run was viewed as "less than."

Since I never ran entire races, I felt like I would never truly fit into that community. I wanted to fit in, but I was never going to be fast, and I most likely would always want to walk some of every race. That underlying sense of judgment separated, in my mind, the running community from the gym community. I had always felt welcomed at the gym by other people in the classes I took, and as I made my way to the free weight section, by the gym members there.

All the while I was running, I thought I was burning a metric ton of calories. I didn't have any fancy watch or monitor back then. I just assumed I was burning a lot of calories because my heart was racing. I was sweating up a storm and it was hard. Really hard. With that logic, I had to be burning a lot of calories, didn't I? This was another reason why running appealed to me. It seemed logical to me at the time, but not having an idea of how many calories I was actually burning ended up being a huge issue.

The reality was I wasn't burning nearly as many calories as I thought. All I knew was I was hungry when I was done, so I ate. A lot. I usually ate high-caloric foods like bagels or energy bars, but also included fruit. As I look back on that time with the wisdom I have now, I can say I was maybe burning three to four hundred calories per run, depending on the length and duration of the run. However, after each run, I ate twice that, most of the time. I was unknowingly spinning my wheels with regards to losing weight. Running was giving me the excuse to eat more. And I did.

You know that saying, "you can't outrun a bad diet?" While my diet wasn't horrific by any means, the concept still applied. It may take you hours to burn four or five hundred calories, but it could take you minutes to consume that many. That, essentially, was what I was doing. For me to eat like that *and* burn enough calories to lose weight through running, I would have to run for longer periods of time daily, and that wasn't feasible. I didn't have that kind of time, nor could my body take that constant pounding, day in and day out. Most importantly, I didn't enjoy it enough. But back then, I still thought if I ran longer races, I would be burning more calories, and eventually I would get the lean look I wanted.

I became intrigued with doing a marathon somewhere along the way. I thought running a marathon was a true test of grit and mental and physical strength. It was something incredibly hard to accomplish, and I thought that was something I wanted to try to do. My next step would be to try a half marathon. In my research, I discovered that Disney World put on several half marathons a year. One of my absolute favorite places to be on this planet—How amazing did that sound? I saw their next half marathon was called the Disney Princess Half Marathon. Everyone dressed up in crazy running costumes. There were Disney characters all along the route. Part of the race went through the Magic Kingdom, and the post-race celebration looked epic. It had my name written all over it. Plus, the course looked really flat, which was another bonus!

Anything Disney does is done exceptionally well, and this race was no exception. Thousands and thousands of people swarmed to Disney World for this race. They had a shuttle system leaving all the Disney Resorts at specified intervals to take the runners to the starting area for the race, starting as early as 3:30 a.m.! Yes, you read that right! Shuttles started that early so they could get everyone to the starting area for the 5 a.m. start time.

Disney races start super early so they can get everyone off the roads, out of the parks, and out of the parking lots before the parks open to the public. I think I must have gotten up at 2 a.m. to get all dolled up in my

Tinkerbell themed costume for the race. My sister-in-law made my skirt out of green netting, which I wore over my running shorts. I also had a green, coordinated tank top and a Tinkerbell baseball hat. I thought I was dressed up a lot—until I saw the people who really dressed up. If nothing else, this race was the best opportunity for people-watching I had ever seen. Some people dressed like Mickey and Minnie, with coordinated shorts or running skirts and matching tops—many with mouse ears. There were also a ton of princesses, running in everything from a t-shirt with their favorite princess to a full-on princess gown. This was obviously not their first rodeo.

I really enjoyed dressing up. My "costume" made me feel like I was truly a part of the race and the whole Disney experience. I have always been a Disney fan, so this was just plain fun in my book.

We didn't have to wait around for a bus—oh no, nothing like that. When I came out of my Disney Resort room and walked to the shuttle pick-up point, there was a line of coaches ready to take everyone to the starting line. There was no waiting. Walk on a bus, and go.

And it was like that at every resort. Typical Disney engineering and efficiency.

Before the race started, they had a huge pre-race festival in a gigantic Disney parking lot. Remember, this is essentially in the middle of the night, but judging from all of the lights, the blaring music, and the hustle and bustle, you would have thought it was a typical outdoor music festival, right down to the rows and rows of portable toilets. Toilets, as far as the eye could see, with lines of people wanting to take their last pee before getting corralled at the start line.

The race crew started herding the runners into their respective starting corrals an hour before race time. My starting block was way in the back. They assign you a block based on your estimated time of finish. The registration form had different time brackets you could check as your estimated finish time. I was looking for the one that said "finish at some point, hopefully still standing up," but as that was not an option, I picked a slow time bracket, which placed me near the back. I literally just wanted to finish. That was it.

By the time my block started the race, my adrenaline was pumping in full force. I was chomping at the bit to just get going, get into whatever rhythm I could find, and take it all in.

As soon as we started, people zoomed by me, weaving in and out. As an inexperienced runner, I started feeling anxious—like I wasn't going fast enough. I started thinking I was for sure going to be last. EVERYONE was passing me (not really, but it felt that way), and I was sure I would be the sole person left on the course.

I had "trained" for this race for months leading up to it. I slowly added mileage to my runs and ran almost eleven miles as my longest run, prior. I did employ the "Run Walk Run" method for most of my training, and it was my intention to do so in this race, but I was getting so anxious at the beginning because everyone was passing me that I kept running, and didn't add in any walking intervals. The voice in the back of my head kept telling me that I was going to end up last, and that I "should be" running the entire time, so I just kept running. I was too jacked up with adrenaline at the start to walk, anyway, and I didn't need to walk that early. Adrenaline was pumping, full force, and I just wanted to go, so I decided to save my walking intervals for when I needed them. Strategically, this sounds smart on the surface—but it sure wasn't smart in reality.

I completely ditched the Run Walk Run methodology at the beginning, and just ran. And kept running. But I eventually did stop. Like, completely stop, because at Disney races, there is a lot to see, even when you are out on the roads running. The race crews set up gigantic floats depicting a scene from a Disney movie, and sometimes they would have costumed characters from that movie there as well. People would hop off the course and stand in line to have their picture taken with whomever was there. It was a lot to see and take in.

This was my kind of race, and they were my kind of people. Runners who didn't take this thing too seriously. Runners who wanted to soak up the entire Disney experience and not just run by it all in a big blur. So I did stop, and stood in a short line to have my picture taken with Woody from Toy Story, because, well…It was Woody. Other than that, I kept plodding along. The Disney race course helped calm my nerves, and really made this race more about having fun and less about having to run a certain pace, or fear finishing last.

As I got well into the race, I started to feel my legs tighten up. A lot. I would literally have to pull off to the side of the course and use a small roller I had brought along with me and stuck in my running fanny pack. My hamstrings were toast. It was at that point that I started the Run Walk Run pattern. This was at about mile eight, out of thirteen.

I eventually crossed the finish line, and my first thought was, *This is the halfway point for a marathon?* I thought there was no way in hell I was ever going to do a marathon. It was probably the quickest decision I have ever made about anything.

It probably sounds like that was my last race, but in fact, it wasn't. I ran two more half marathons soon after that one. After you accomplish something that you never really thought you could do, you get a wave of confidence. While I didn't think full marathons would be in my future, I had so much fun at the Disney race that I entered another Disney Race the next year, and a few months after that, another half marathon that was closer to home.

I had the honor of meeting Jeff Galloway, the creator of Run Walk Run, at the Run Disney Expo before my second Disney half marathon. I told him how my first race went, how miserable my hamstrings were as a result, and how the walking didn't seem to help me much.

After he graciously listened to me, he said to me, "Susan (with a grand pause), my guess is you didn't start your Run Walk Run intervals until much later in the race, am I correct?"

I looked sheepishly at him and replied, "Yes, that is exactly what happened"

Ugh, I was caught!

He guaranteed that if I employed the method from the very beginning, even though I didn't feel like I needed it, I would have a much different experience this time around.

And boy, was he right. My second half marathon experience was totally different from the first. I started my Run Walk Run intervals immediately after I started, and I crossed the finish line in one piece, able to not only walk afterward, but run. What a difference listening to instructions and checking your ego at the door can make!

While I enjoyed the fun part of the races (being at Disney, the Expo, the course, the characters, and the after-race party), if I am being truly honest here, I still didn't enjoy running.

I found it extremely challenging. I was a heavy runner, meaning I was not light on my feet—and I am certain my stride left a lot to be desired. I found running liberating, from the perspective of being able to put on your shoes and go, no equipment needed. I also found running to be very challenging, mentally, which was tough to conquer. The first few miles were torture on the brain. So many times, I wanted to quit before I actually got going. Running included maybe the toughest mental challenge of any physical activity I had done up to that point. But in all honesty, running did nothing for my weight loss or my physique. I didn't realize, at the time, how much I used running as a justification for overeating.

So once again, I was spinning my wheels, doing something I didn't really enjoy all that much.

I am sure if I had gotten a running coach who worked with me on my gait, pace, different types of running workouts, and so on, it might have been different—but running ended up not being for me.

I enjoyed the thought of running more than I enjoyed running itself. But there was something on the horizon that I was about to get hooked on, something that had been piquing my interest every time I went to the gym: strength training.

CHAPTER 5
HOW LIFTING BECAME MY PASSION

I got a taste of strength training back in the nineties. I was always fascinated by the free weight section, and how hard people there seemed to be working. They all looked strong, and that was very appealing to me. At first, I was introduced to the basic machines and dumbbells. I don't remember using a barbell, although I probably did squat with a barbell at one time or another. The gym I belonged to was less of a powerlifting or crossfit gym, and more of a typical big box gym: lots of machines, lots of free weights, and lots and lots of cardio equipment.

Training back then was very different than it is today. The overall emphasis was far more focused on cardio-based exercise. The aerobics craze was in full swing, and the benefits of strength training for the average person (as opposed to body builders) wasn't talked about. Weights seemed to only be something for the big guys/bros. Women tended to only be in the aerobics classes and on the cardio machines.

Truth is, strength training was never just for young men. It was and always will be beneficial to anyone, of any gender and at any age. Becoming stronger and building muscle is essential for living a healthy and functional life, especially as you get older. We lose muscle as we age, we lose bone density as we age, and we lose strength as we age. But the great news is that strength training can turn all of that around. I like to call it the true Fountain of Youth.

I was attracted to strength training. Lifting heavy stuff and being strong was something that was more appealing to me than jumping around off beat to music.

I remember watching people in the free weight section of the weight room, where there were racks and racks of dumbbells. It was the area where all the "bros" hung out—younger guys who were big, muscular and lifted a ton of weight.

That area was intimidating to me. It interested me, but I didn't want to go in there. I was afraid of people looking at me, judging me, making fun of me, all of it. I didn't really know what I was doing, but I did eventually muster the courage to go over there and "lift some weight."

One of my first times venturing into the weight section, I grabbed a pair of dumbells (DBs) and did what I thought was a chest exercise: basically holding DBs out to the sides with my elbows at ninety degrees (I called that scarecrow arms), and moving the DBs in toward the center of my chest and back out.

I'm not sure why I was doing that. I had no idea what it was for, really. My initial thought was that it was a chest exercise, so it must be good, right? I probably did it because I had seen it in a class or in some fitness magazine—but more realistically, I did it because I had no plan and no idea what to do. After I had finished a couple reps of whatever I was doing, some random guy came up to me and told me I was basically doing nothing. I wasn't really working on anything.

My biggest fear of going into the weight room had just been realized. Even though the guy was really kind to me, I was embarrassed. I had definitely been looked at, and I thought I had been judged

While now I can appreciate his candor with me, back then he almost brought my strength training journey to a screeching halt before it really began. I was humiliated, and if I am being brutally honest here, I probably didn't venture back to that part of the gym for a while. I stuck to those classes I knew and felt safe in, the aerobics classes with some light weight training at the end. They were fun, and most importantly (to me at the time), they were a safe environment.

I was really intimidated to go back into that weight room. I could have allowed that intimidation to keep me from ever going back, and from ever learning how to get stronger. If I gave in to my fear, I could have avoided it forever.

When we avoid something out of fear, it's usually some fear that we have made up in our head, like, "What if people stare at me?" or, "What if people laugh at me?" or, "What if I mess up an exercise?"

All those questions aren't reality, in the vast majority of scenarios.

We always think that people are staring at us and judging us in the gym, when the reality is they aren't. Most people in the gym are focused on what they are doing, not what someone else is doing. They don't give a rat's ass what you are doing. They want to get on with their workout and go home.

And what if there is that single asshole in the gym who might be staring or saying something? Well, so what? There are always jerks in this world—there's no way to avoid them—but the vast majority of people in gyms are not jerks at all.

That said, if you encounter one, keep this in mind: are you going to let one jerk keep you from reaching your goals?

Absolutely not.

The only way to attack any fear is to deal with it head on. There are many different angles you can hit it from. What I opted to do to help build my confidence was to hire a trainer who could guide me, teach me appropriate exercises, and hold me accountable.

I recommend anyone who is just starting out in the strength training world to hire a trainer at your gym, even if it's just for a handful of sessions. Have someone there to teach you the basics and make sure you are performing the exercises correctly. You will develop a confidence that will carry you forward into not only the weight room, but into every other aspect of your life.

It's like opening the floodgates. Once a little confidence starts, you will see everything change. It's really fun to watch my clients, who started off unsure and intimidated, to lift heavier weight. They gradually build confidence and want to lift even more weight, and then I get to see how that bleeds over into every other aspect of their lives.

Maybe they will feel confident enough to take a class in an area that is way out of their expertise. Maybe they will go back to school. Maybe they will finally leave their job where they have been miserable for so long.

I've seen it all.

After that failed attempt at a "chest exercise," I decided that since I really was that clueless as to what to do in the free weight section, I needed some guidance. That was the final nudge I needed to hire a trainer and start learning.

As I mentioned in chapter 3, I hired David who taught me a ton. He was super patient, and I was super eager to learn. I started getting stronger, and I loved that. There was something about feeling strong that I loved. Maybe it was me developing sense of confidence that was starting to show. I seemed to carry myself differently, and I started to feel like an athlete of sorts. I felt like I was getting good at it.

Getting strong is addictive, folks. It's unlike any other feeling. It doesn't matter how old you are; strength has no age requirement. Everyone will benefit from getting stronger.

Getting stronger will improve your daily functional life, including: sitting, standing, picking up heavy things without hurting your back, picking up your grandkids, strengthening your joints so you can move without pain, and so much more. And, best of all, you'll get to watch how that improvement transfers over into every other aspect of your life.

Don't let gym intimidation or the lack of knowledge on what to do be the reason you don't strength train. Take control, get some help, and start building strength. Your life will change dramatically—for the better.

After I had my baby, I was forced to change gyms. We had moved to a neighboring town, and going back and forth to the old gym with a newborn at home wasn't working, so my time with David had to come to an end. But I vowed to continue my journey at my new gym, with a new trainer.

I found a gym very close to my home and I gave it a try. I had been walking and trying to eat "healthy," but was ready to get back into the gym. I received some free training sessions as a new member, but the trainer who I was working with really didn't know what to do with me. He was a very nice young man, but I honestly think my post-pregnancy" condition" made him uncomfortable. In some odd way, I felt sorry for him. We didn't click at all, so our trainer/client relationship didn't last too long.

That particular gym wasn't a great environment, either. It was full of lots of big dudes who got to a squat rack and kept it occupied for long periods of time, and as a new mom, I didn't have thirty minutes or more to sit and wait for a squat rack to open up; I had to get home. I never liked the vibe, and I never really felt comfortable there, so my relationship with that particular gym soon came to a screeching halt.

I eventually found a gym that had child care on site, so once Mike became old enough, I became a regular there. I could take him with me and not have to worry about getting someone to watch him while I went to the gym. It definitely took a lot of pressure off, but it wasn't all smooth sailing.

There were many times where one of the child care workers would come out and interrupt my workout because Mike threw up, or I forgot a diaper, or something like that. And I know that many of you might be thinking, "Eww! Those child care places are so dirty, why would you even take your child there?" I was never one of those Moms who got overly worried about stuff like that. Maybe I should have been, but I just wasn't. Mike was a healthy kid, and I figured he was going to get his fair share of childhood illnesses at some point—there was no stopping it—so I didn't see a need to be overprotective with stuff like that. He survived just fine.

Over the course of about fifteen years, I worked with many different trainers, all of whom taught me a great deal about exercises and technique, and I'm super grateful to each and every one of them.

However, one thing that was missing from all the trainers was any kind of nutrition plan. Back in the day, most nutrition help came from going to Weight Watchers, Jenny Craig, or seeing a dietician. Not a single one of the trainers I ever worked with talked to me about how weight loss actually *worked*, like how you need to be in a calorie deficit and what that even meant, how starving yourself wasn't the long-term solution, or how to develop a sustainable way of eating.

None of that ever happened.

So while my love of strength training was growing, my nutrition education was not. I was starting to see the strength gains, which I loved, but I wasn't leaning out like I wanted. Even so, I kept on. In my mind, I was thinking, "If I just work a little bit harder, I'll lose the weight I want to lose."

What I didn't realize at the time was that, without any nutritional guidance, I would just continue to spin my wheels.

Working with trainers was something I loved. One particular trainer really lit a fire in me. He was smart and always pushing me, and I started to really feel like I was strong. As I mentioned, feeling strong is unlike anything else. You start to carry yourself differently; you start to speak up more. And for the first time, I started thinking that maybe this was something I should pursue. I was a school counselor at the time, and I loved working out, so what could be a better marriage? I loved to talk to people and help people, and I loved to work out, so I decided I would get certified as a trainer myself.

However, while I wanted to get certified, I was still having an internal struggle with Yo-Yo dieting myself. I was still in a pattern of losing and gaining weight—but somewhere deep inside, I kept thinking getting certified would not only help me with that struggle, but also give me the opportunity to really help people with their training.

I got certified by The American Council on Exercise (ACE), one of the most well-respected certifications in the industry, after completing an at-home study course.

My music and psychology background didn't prepare me for the first chapter in the book. It was all anatomy, and I got very intimidated. I almost quit before I started, as it was way out of my comfort zone, but I decided to dive in and go old school.

I made a TON of note cards. One thing I have learned over the years is that when you write things down (as opposed to typing), you retain more of what you are writing, so I took the time to create note cards on everything—not only the anatomy section, but the entire book.

There were many online study groups and webinars that I participated in to help prepare for the final exam. There were also CDs you could listen to in the car that went over information as well. The educator in me completely loved how they were trying to tap into different learning styles: audio, visual, and reading. They covered a lot of bases and I tried it all, but being the old-school person I was, in-person learning was really my jam.

Despite all the studying, in all honesty, I was struggling. Doing all this on my own was a massive undertaking. I was trying to balance studying on my own with being a mom, having a full-time job, and keeping up my own workout schedule. I was still trying to get in five or six workouts a week, and I was still in the same nutrition mode of eating fairly clean with little to no regard to calories.

Previously I had gone back to school for my masters degree in School Counseling. It was a way different experience. Education was in a field I was very familiar with. Even though some of the counseling content was new, the overarching content was very familiar, and all the course work was in person, not online. This new way of learning was very challenging for me.

Eventually I saw that ACE was hosting an in-person study seminar for those who were preparing to take the exam. It was a two-day event, where an ACE instructor walked us through everything we needed to know for the test. We had the opportunity to ask questions and collaborate with other people who were preparing to take the exam as well.

This was exactly what I needed: Being in a classroom with other people and not in front of a computer screen, and being able to ask questions to a live human being and have a meaningful discussion. I left there feeling more confident and more prepared than I had been at any time during this process. I was ready.

I scheduled the exam as soon as I got home. I went to the testing center a few weeks later to take the timed exam, and I passed with flying colors!

I was a Personal Trainer, certified by one of the most respected groups in the fitness industry. I was incredibly excited and nervous all at the same time to officially be a member of the Trainer community. The next chapter of my life had begun.

CHAPTER 6

WORKING OUT: TOO MUCH OF A GOOD THING?

As my training continued, my love of lifting was growing even stronger. I was in the gym six or seven days a week, working hard. Unfortunately, all the working out didn't show, from a weight loss perspective. I hadn't made any real significant changes to how I looked. Translation: I hadn't lost much, if any, fat.

I was still trying to eat healthy, but I was not paying close attention to quantity, and—as I would learn—quantity is what will drive your weight loss.

I began working with another trainer who pushed me even more, and a couple times, I did two workouts in a day. At the time, that sounded amazing to me.

When I did those workouts, it was not a lifting session and then later a cardio session, it was usually two lifting sessions. Cardio was not on my radar anymore. Running was in the rearview mirror. I would occasionally walk on a treadmill, or maybe even run some intervals, but nothing more than that. Lifting was what I wanted to do.

And the two-a-days? I started out loving them. I pushed myself super super hard in each session. Looking back, the plan I was given was not well thought out at all, but I didn't know that then. All I knew was I was going to the gym twice in a day on some days, and I loved it. I loved the feeling of working hard, and I loved gaining strength. If working out two times a day would help me get stronger, then sign me up!

It took its toll, though. I was exhausted, I wasn't sleeping well, and I was sore a lot—not only sore; my body was physically drained. It was hard to move, sometimes. I was zapped of energy. I was on the fast track to burning out. I wasn't giving my body a chance to recover, and it was starting to show. But through it all, I still loved every single second. Since I thought more equaled better, I figured that the more I worked out, the better I would get. Sounds logical, right? The more I worked out, the stronger I would get, and the leaner I would become. All sounds great on the surface, but it's not how it works.

I would often get asked, "Susan, why are you working out so much?" My standard answer was always the same: Because I love it.

This is what I told everyone. I loved working out. It was something I felt I was becoming good at, and something that I really enjoyed, so I was speaking the truth.

But here's the thing. That wasn't the *entire* truth. I did love it, and I still love it, but if I was being truly honest, I would have said: I workout so much because I'm afraid.

- I'm afraid if I don't work out this much, I will lose progress.
- I am afraid if I don't work out this much, I won't make any more progress.
- Worst of all, I am afraid if I don't work out this much, I will remain fat and never actually lose the weight.

That was the real truth. I lived in fear.

I felt like I had to workout that hard all the time, or all of my biggest fears would come to reality. I would sometimes even add a little extra cardio. I was using these little mini-bouts of cardio to burn extra calories on top of whatever else I had done that day. If the treadmill told me I burned three hundred calories, that was amazing. I wasn't tracking calories, so I really had no clue as to exactly what that number meant in terms of food, but in my head, it made me feel like I had things under control.

As I've said, those numbers the treadmill, elliptical, and fitness watch tell you about how many calories you've burned are inherently wrong—sometimes as much as fifty percent wrong. The Stanford University School of Medicine conducted a study in 2017 that showed out of seven devices tested, none showed accurate calorie expenditure. The most accurate device was off by 27% and the least accurate device was off by 93%. If your treadmill, or your watch says you burned four hundred calories, it's probably more like 250-275. So when you eat an additional four hundred calories (probably more) to celebrate a job well done...well, do you see the problem? You have just put yourself in the "plus" column for calories, instead of being in a deficit. You have added calories back into your diet that you didn't burn.

This is a big problem for a lot of people. I see it all the time. My best advice? Ignore those numbers, from whatever source you use. None of them are accurate enough for you to be able to reliably add those calories back in and assure yourself you will be in a deficit. Not even your really expensive fitness watch or tracker is accurate enough.

But I didn't know any of this at the time, so in my mind, those numbers gave me a false sense of accomplishment.

At the gym, where I was working out, I started to figure out that a particular treadmill's numbers would be higher than the others. It would tell me I was burning more calories than the other treadmills would, so there would be occasions where I would actually wait to get on that specific treadmill (if it was in use) because it would make me feel even more accomplished.

When I write this down, it sounds absolutely crazy. I would wait for a treadmill because it would give more favorable information than the others would, not realizing that none of those numbers, whether they were from that one particular treadmill or any other treadmill, were even close to being accurate. Waiting for a specific treadmill should have been my red flag, but it wasn't. I just wanted to see those higher numbers.

That's what fear will do to you. It will take all logic and common sense out of the equation.

The best thing you can do is focus on what you can control, not output numbers from machines or different pieces of technology. Focus on what you consume, because that is what you ultimately can control. Yes, those calories burned will count and help with weight loss, but you won't know exactly how many you are burning. Consider any calories that you are burning along the way as an additional contributor to the calorie deficit you have created with your nutrition. I like to call burned calories a bonus, or even "extra credit." Deprogram the feature from your watch or machine that tells you how many calories you burned. Don't even look at the numbers. Just do your thing, and keep the deficit calorie number the same.

So as you can imagine, I was making zero progress. My lifts weren't increasing, I was tired all the time, I was dragging myself to the gym, and I started to get some injuries along the way

I had in my mind that more was better. The more I did, the better my results would be. If I had 3 sets I would do 4. If I had 10 reps I would do 15. That's how I was thinking. More is better.

Another news flash: more is not better. *Better* is better. Making your current workouts more effective by increasing weight, slowing your reps down, and focusing on technique are great ways to make what you are doing more effective. Weight training is about the quality you bring to the workout, not about how many workouts you do.

All of my fears were completely irrational, yet I kept doing the same thing over and over, expecting a different result. According to Einstein, that is the actual definition of insanity. I had allowed my emotions to dictate what I was doing, and that is always a big recipe for disaster.

As a coach, I see this all the time. Every single day, I talk to people who are struggling to lose fat or keep it off, and the first thing out of their mouths is usually about how much they are working out.

"I work out six days a week, and run three days a week. I add a kickboxing class once a week, and I am thinking about adding in a Bootcamp once a week," they tell me, all in one breath.

When I ask them why they are working out so much, I get a really familiar answer: "Because I just love it!"

I can almost recite exactly how our conversation is going to go. Sometimes they get angry with me along the way, because I would hit a nerve—one that I wish someone had hit with me, way back when. People don't like to be challenged. I get that. It's incredibly difficult to be honest with yourself. It's way easier to gloss over the truth and just keep spinning your wheels. Change can be scary.

Having a coach to challenge you in that way can be scary and frustrating, but life-changing. Changing your mindset is not like flipping a switch—it is tough, and takes practice over time. It takes practice to shut down the voices in your head that are saying you have to work out six or seven days a week in order to make progress. It takes practice to be honest with yourself with what you are doing—and, more importantly, why you are doing it.

As soon as we can be honest with ourselves about what is happening, as soon as we stop allowing our emotions to dictate what we do, we can get out of the hamster wheel we have been stuck in for (in my case) decades and finally start to make some progress.

Look: you don't have to workout six or seven days a week. In fact, you're better off not working out that much, because you are leaving out probably *the* most important aspect of training, the part where all the strength and muscle gains occur: rest days.

I don't think most people understand the power of rest days. And I mean real rest days, not days where you go for a "light" five-mile run, but days where you may go for a walk, stretch, or better yet, do nothing and actually allow your body to rest. Those days are when the gains happen.

When you lift weights, you are tearing up your muscle fibers. Literally, you are creating microscopic tears in your muscles. Rest days allow your muscles and connective tissue to repair and rebuild. Rest days also allow your central nervous system to recover, and when you allow your body to do these things, your next workout will be way more effective.

You will have more energy for your lifts, and you will build muscle and strength more effectively.

Rest is an essential part of building muscle and strength. Without rest, you will be exercising a body that is in need of recovery, and you could be headed toward injuries—which is exactly what happened to me.

If you are feeling emotionally drained from hitting so hard so often, rest days will also allow your brain to decompress, relax, and recover, as well.

Rest doesn't have to mean lying around all day. It can mean going for a walk or a bike ride, a more "active" rest. But adding a short high-intensity circuit or another short workout does not constitute rest.

As a coach, I talk about the importance of rest days all the time. None of my previous trainers ever did that for me. The mentality seemed to be to "go big or go home," back then. There was no real guidance with regards to rest days and how important they actually are in your training.

What was also missing, as I mentioned, was the lack of nutrition guidance.

CHAPTER 7
GOOD VS. BAD FOOD MENTALITY

I have come to despise the words "eating clean." It is a term I used for many years. I think it was one of those trendy terms. "Oh, I eat clean." That must mean I am doing something good, right?

I don't even know what that means anymore, primarily because "clean" can mean something different to every person. For one person it can mean eating all organic foods, while to another it could mean going completely vegan.

I used this term, "eating clean," for years and years. It was like a badge of honor. For me, eating clean meant I only ate foods that were considered "healthy." This meant whole, unprocessed, healthy foods. I wasn't big into the "organic" thing, though. I didn't see the benefits then and, honestly, that may have been the one thing I was on target with. I have learned that, in most cases, organic isn't worth the extra money.. Organic does allow the use of some pesticides, and organic doesn't mean unprocessed which many think it means. All food is processed to some degree or other unless it is coming directly from your backyard. Buying and eating organic foods won't hurt anything for sure, but I could just never bring myself to pay the extra money.

Here is a list of what I would eat when I was eating clean:

- Protein - a large variety of meats (Yes, even red meats)
- Vegetables - all different kinds
- Fruit - especially avocados
- Nuts and nut butters - I loved nuts
- Olive oil - used for everything
- Whole grains - whole grain pasta, whole grain breads, whole grain rice, etc.

If it didn't have the word "whole," I probably didn't eat it.

Looks great on the surface, doesn't it? These are all foods that most people would consider healthy, and they are mostly nutrient dense. So, what's the problem? Can't go wrong there, right?

Well, there were a few problems.

The first problem was that it was a very small circle of foods. I wasn't allowing myself to enjoy much of anything outside of that circle. There were plenty of other foods I loved, like pizza, hamburgers, French fries, donuts, and chocolate cake, but I thought if I allowed any of those foods in my diet, in *any* amount, I would ruin whatever progress I had made because those were "bad" foods.

Having those foods was asking for trouble in my book, so I avoided them completely.

And so, my "good" versus "bad" food philosophy began.

My relationship with these "good" and "bad" foods was tumultuous at best, and it resulted in me putting a ton of pressure on myself, my family, and my friends.

Trying to dodge all of the "bad" foods led me to avoid (or wanting to avoid) social situations that would include those foods. I was not equipped to handle any kind of curve ball to my normal routine and my normal circle of foods. So when my family wanted to go out for dinner, they always asked me to choose where we could go that would have something I could actually eat.

I think they viewed me as a picky eater, and I guess I was, but never thought of it that way. I just viewed it as trying to be "healthy."

I was beginning to feel like my diet was overly restrictive, but I thought this was the only way to go.

My family were all absolute angels for putting up with that for so long. They wanted to support me, and that was one way they were attempting to show it. But how narrow-minded and obsessed does that situation sound?

I truly thought if I went to a restaurant and had a burger and fries, I would ruin all the progress I had made. I didn't understand that one meal is not going to ruin progress. It is impossible to gain fat from just one meal, but I didn't understand that.

And you know what the real irony of that is? I was making zero progress, when it came to my weight, anyway. None.

But in my head, I thought I was doing everything right. Praising the nutritious foods, and demonizing the less nutritious foods, all the while keeping to my restricted food bubble.

And to top it all off, I was miserable.

Some may say that my food bubble was not "that" small, or "that" restrictive, and they would be right—as long as I stayed in my own house and had complete control over what I ate.

But that is no way to live.

When I worked as a school counselor, we had office birthday parties. We would each bring in some treats and goodies for their birthday, and then we would all gather in the office kitchen, sing Happy Birthday, and celebrate. Typically, people would bring in cupcakes or a cake of some kind. Sometimes people would even bring in breakfast items, which would include pastries, bagels, donuts, things like that. And on every single birthday I never took part in the treats. I would be in the room to celebrate with the person, I would sing Happy Birthday, I would sign the card, and I would give them all of my good wishes, but I would *never* partake in the treats that were brought in. Even when I brought in treats for someone else's birthday, I didn't eat anything that I brought in, myself.

They would pass around cupcakes and I would say, "No, thank you." They would pass around a piece of cake and I would say, "No, thank you." And everyone kept telling me, "Susan, you are so disciplined. I wish I could be like you."

And while they were thinking that and telling me that, I was thinking to myself, "*I* want to be like *you*. I want to be able to enjoy a cupcake. I am dying to have a piece of that chocolate cake. I want to be able to participate!"

I felt like I was in prison.

On the outside, it looked like I was being disciplined, but on the inside, I was dying. I would tell everyone that I was full, or that it would make my stomach feel bad later, or that I just didn't want the cupcake. That was a bold-faced lie. I wanted the cupcake, and more than that I wanted the freedom to choose whether I took the cupcake or not. I didn't feel like I had that freedom, because my fear of the cupcake ruining my progress was so great.

But the more people told me how disciplined I was, the more it fueled the fire, and the more it gave me the false belief that I was, indeed, being disciplined

I loved being called "disciplined!" It made me feel like I was not only doing the right thing, but the hard thing. The thing others wished they could do but couldn't. Yet, I could. In some weird way, it was a sign of strength.

Yet, if you reverse the roles, it was exactly the same in *my* eyes. Everyone else was strong, because they could allow themselves to have that cupcake, and I couldn't, because when I did have the cupcake or the piece of cake, the guilt would eat me alive.

One time, it was my own birthday, and I declined a piece of my *own* birthday cake. Everyone else was enjoying the cake that was brought in for me, and I was just standing there, being appreciative and wishing I could go hide. Previously, I always had a piece of my own cake, but that one time I just couldn't do it. I am not sure why that particular birthday was so different, but it was. I fumbled around excuses like, "I had a big birthday lunch and I am stuffed! But I will take the cake home and enjoy it with my family later." I took the cake home and my husband and son would eat most of it. I cut the tiniest sliver of cake, so tiny that it was almost impossible to cut.

That was probably a new low for me. I felt like a complete failure, and I was humiliated. I promised myself, that day, that I would never turn down my own birthday cake again. And I kept that promise.

Back then, I wasn't "disciplined" at all. I was overly restrictive. Eating "clean" was such a badge of honor back then that it had taken over my existence. People admired my ability to pass up on the "bad" foods, but they didn't see how miserable that restriction made me feel on the inside.

The whole "good" food versus "bad" food idea is such a slippery slope. The more we categorize food that way, the more you are opening yourself up to overly restricting, bingeing, and developing a poor relationship with food.

Food is just food. Some foods have more calories than others, and some foods are more nutrient dense than others, but in the big picture, food is just food. The problem comes in when you think you can't have certain foods because they are "bad" (higher in calories, less nutrition dense). You have to realize that living life means enjoying foods of all different types, not just the "good" foods.

Have you ever done any of these after eating a food you might consider "bad"?

- Beat yourself up for "giving in"
- Binge on those foods because you have restricted them for so long
- Feel guilty and ashamed
- Do extra bouts of cardio as a punishment

This is where the poor relationship with food comes in, and how it starts to affect aspects of your life. The thought of going off track is enough to instill panic around situations where you might encounter those "bad" foods, so you start opting out of social gatherings.

That's a big line to cross.

We all should aim to eat mostly nutrient dense foods as the majority of our diet for optimum health, but understanding that you can (and I would go as far to say should) include "fun" foods into your diet, all while remaining healthy and on track to reaching your weight loss goals is key to sustainability.

Jordan Syatt, world-record holder powerlifter and owner of Syatt Fitness, did a thirty-day challenge where he ate a Big Mac every single day for thirty days. He lost seven pounds. How did he do it? He planned. He counted the calories from the Big Mac and included it in his overall daily calorie amount. The rest of his daily calories came from lean protein, vegetables, and fruit. The point of this challenge was to show that you can include any food in your diet that you want, and you can still lose weight, as long as you make it work.

This is not to imply that you should eat a Big Mac, or any other similar food, every day. That challenge just showed that it is, in fact, possible to include foods you love within your diet and still lose weight.

The biggest takeaway? Weight loss does not have to be about the complete elimination of any food or food group.

So, how do we do it? How do we actually lose weight?

CHAPTER 8
LOSING FAT: WHAT REALLY WORKS

Over the years, things in the fitness and diet world changed and evolved, which made things even more complicated. It seemed like one year it was all about low fat, and how fat was what made you fat. Then later, it was all about no carbs, and how carbs were the devil and *they* were what was making you fat.

It's no wonder we are all confused.

However, there is one thing that has held true over every diet, has stood the test of time, and is what actually works: being in a calorie deficit.

Eat fewer calories than your body needs. That's how you lose weight.

It is pretty simple in concept, but knowing how to actually do it is where the problems can begin. One of the biggest mistakes I see is exactly what I did: becoming overly restrictive.

For a period of time, I used a SlimFast Shake as a meal replacement, along with a Ziplock of Cheerios. I wanted to keep what I ate to minimum, and thought that was a great way to have control. But what I didn't think about was the sustainability factor. Was this a viable way to keep calories in control over the long haul? Was this even a way of eating that I wanted to keep doing forever? Those kinds of questions are important to ask yourself when you embark on a diet or a new way of eating. If the answer is no, then you should find a different way of eating that you will be able to sustain over time.

I didn't think about those questions at all. Big mistake.

SlimFast and Cheerios didn't work well for me. It didn't fill me up (no real surprise there) and as a result the nibbling would begin. Almonds were a go-to healthy snack for me. And make no mistake, almonds are a great source of fats (not protein—too little protein for the amount of calories), but they are also calorie dense. So those two or three handfuls of almonds I would have to take the edge off my hunger would probably add over 400 calories to my daily intake, which didn't even include any of the numerous little bites, tastes, and other things I didn't even notice I ate throughout the day

Back then, I wasn't tracking or thinking about calories. I was only thinking about eating "clean" or eating healthy, and I was telling myself that if the foods were healthy, quantity wasn't important. One cupcake would ruin me, but a whole bag of almonds was perfectly fine. To me, quality was way more important. And let's be clear: while they are both important, quantity rules the roost if you want to lose fat.

Let me repeat that: quantity of calories rules when it comes to fat loss.

So, not understanding this, I paid no attention to the quantity (calories) of anything that I ate. Remember how my family would only go out to places I deemed "clean" and "healthy" enough for me? My favorite restaurant back then was a little hole-in-the-wall, family-owned place that we frequented almost every week.

My go-to meal there was a grilled chicken and pasta dish. Doesn't sound too bad, right? It had grilled chicken, which of course was way healthier than fried chicken, and some kind of "whole this" or "whole that" pasta with pesto. In my mind, that made it a healthy dish.

The dish would arrive in a ginormous bowl. There was no marinara or alfredo, or anything like that, just the pesto and whatever oils were used in preparation. This was another reason why I considered this dish a great healthy choice. But the bowl was huge.

I literally ate the entire bowl. Yes, the entire bowl, every time, never thinking twice about it. Looking back on it, I probably consumed almost 1500 calories, just in that one dish.

And the irony here is that I picked that restaurant and that pasta dish because I assumed it was "good" for me. All 1500+ calories of it.

I was doing myself zero favors.

But that was how skewed my view of nutrition was. Eating healthy was the way to go, no matter how much I ate. But there was a subconscious theme going on in the back of my mind back then that, looking back, was the driving force behind me not wanting to explore nutrition more, or change anything else I was doing.

I was afraid.

Just like my fear of scaling back my training, I was afraid to look into my nutrition beyond a fleeting glance. I was afraid of what I would learn. I was afraid to find out how many calories that grilled chicken and pasta dish had. I was afraid to know how many calories the almonds contained. I didn't want to know. Ignorance was bliss.

The fear of learning about all of that would mean I would be faced with change. And I wasn't ready for that (or, I didn't think I was, anyway). I had also made up my mind that any kind of tracking or counting calories was going to take the joy out of eating and out of my life in general, so I wasn't about to do that. I just stayed on the hamster wheel that I knew, thinking that it would eventually work out at some point

I was wrong.

I was stuck. Not making any progress, but afraid to change anything. It's fascinating to look back, because it makes no sense. I was not making any progress whatsoever, yet I kept doing the exact same thing over and over and over again.

This is a great example of allowing emotions to make your decisions. The exact same scenario that played out with my training was playing out with my nutrition. The emotion in control was, again, fear. I was afraid of what I would find out if I really dove into what I was doing. The biggest part of that fear? Feeling like a complete failure yet again.

The biggest fear for a Yo-Yo dieter is failing. You live with that fear every single day. You want so badly to get out of the Yo-Yo cycle, and to be able to finally conquer what has been haunting you for so many years, but you defy any and all logic, and stay right where you are: in the hamster wheel of frustration, feeling like you will never get out.

It was the same type of fear that kept me working out so much. An illogical fear that if I didn't keep up the workout pace I had, I would lose progress, and gain fat.

I didn't want to feel humiliated. I didn't want to admit I didn't have this thing down.

As a coach, I often see people who know what to do, but just aren't doing it. I also see a lot of people who think they are doing everything they need to do, but in reality, they aren't. The latter was me.

We are in an age where we can get information right at our fingertips. We can access anything in a matter of seconds, which sounds like a good thing. Some may argue that too much information can muddy the waters, but I truly believe that *most* people do, in fact, know what to do:
- Eat mostly nutrient-dense foods
- Keep portions reasonable

- Allow yourself some treats along the way
- Move every day

There are many ways to fine-tune the above, but that's the basic template. We all logically know this, so why can't we be consistent with it, or even do it at all?

I truly don't think it's laziness or lack of motivation or anything similar. I think that, for some of us, our belief in ourselves to be able to accomplish goals is a huge player. We doubt our ability to succeed, our self-efficacy.

My self-efficacy ebbed and flowed depending on where I was in my Yo-Yo cycle. If my weight was down, my confidence and self-efficacy were fairly high, but they would plummet when the weight slowly came back.

Somewhere along the way, maybe through life events or muddling through tough times, we start to doubt our ability to succeed. Phrases like, "That doesn't work for me," or, "I could never do that," start to pop up in our vocabulary and become our go-to. Those phrases become a shield. Those phrases become our excuses. Our reasons why we aren't making progress. And we actually start to believe them, because it's way easier to believe something doesn't work for you than it is to dig in and put in the work. Essentially, they protect us from failure. They are another way of saying, "I don't think I can do this, so I am going to lay the groundwork for failure to protect me." When we do this enough, before we know it, we have stripped ourselves of confidence and the belief that we can actually succeed.

So, my career as a Yo-Yo dieter continued. It involved periods of restricting "bad" foods and overeating "healthy" foods as well as some diets that were cleverly marketed as the best way to finally lose weight, and lose it FAST.

I went through some of them and lived to tell about it! In addition to Jenny Craig and the SlimFast period, I tried some of the craziest diets of the day like going completely fat free (because fat was the devil), and stuck my feet in the water of Atkins (super low carb), but I love carbs too much for that.

The irony about these diets is that they could *all* work. You can lose weight on every single one of them, if you are in a calorie deficit. But, sustaining and maintaining that weight loss is an entirely different story. Most of these diets eliminate entire macro groups, or specific foods with no real exit plan. Most people can sustain a very restrictive diet for a short period of time, but embracing that way of eating forever is not what most people want to do.

One thing I have learned over the years of trying fad diets is that on these diets, success is temporary. If the plan you are on is not inclusive and preaching sustainability, you most likely will not be able to adopt it as a lifestyle.

Have you ever said anything like, "I am going back to {insert name of diet here} because {diet} works for me."

If you constantly have to go back to it, is it, in fact, "working for you?"

I always like to ask my clients this question when they start talking about different diets: Can you see yourself eating like this for the rest of your life?

If the answer is no, then why would you even do it?

So throughout this Yo-Yo time, my eating, for the most part, didn't change much, and my fat and skinny clothes were still around. I made brief, failed attempts at some novel way of overly restricting food, was not able to keep it up, then punished myself with a million crunches after I ate too much. Ultimately, I felt like this was how it was always going to be.

So on I went. Doing the same thing, with no sustainable results. And as I continued on into my forties and fifties, I ran head-on into my friend. Her name is Menopause.

CHAPTER 9
DIET, TRAINING, AND MENOPAUSE

Getting old is not for the faint of heart, and that includes going through menopause. I didn't know much about menopause at all. In fact, I didn't know *anything*, really. I find it interesting that menopause is not a subject that is talked about a lot. It is not a subject that even your doctors talk about very much. It seems like the only way you ever learn about menopause is if you dig deep and start researching it for yourself. Digging deep and researching for yourself sounds great, but not many people have the time to dig through all of the articles, blog posts, and research that there is out there.

I am happy to say that in the last several years, menopause has been brought to the forefront more, especially in the fitness community. Myself and my colleagues are talking about menopause, our experiences, what the research says, and bringing an awareness to it, with the purpose of demystifying the subject. These kinds of discussions are literally helping women all over the world. There are so many assumptions about menopause that are just completely wrong, and we are trying to spread the truth and give women hope.

And the biggest hope of them all is: you can, in fact, still lose weight, and build some muscle, while in menopause—or even after menopause.

This bears repeating: it's never too late to lose weight and build muscle.

When I went through menopause, I didn't really know what was happening. All I knew was that I had weird, unexplained physical symptoms, and some of those symptoms were pretty severe. I had tingling in my left arm, vertigo-type sensations, and unexplained extreme malaise, just to name a few. It became difficult to function for an entire day at my school.

After a little while of this, I committed the ultimate sin of looking up my symptoms on WebMD. Big mistake. You can literally look up any symptoms on WebMD and think you are dying, so my low-level anxiety was starting to climb fast.

I went to my general practitioner and specialists, several times. No one seemed to have any answers. For a while, I thought I had a heart problem, Multiple Sclerosis (MS), or some other neurological disorder, but no one seemed to know.

I ended up with my ENT, who said he found "something." He found some (very little) damage to my inner ear, with no real explanation as to why. He didn't seem one hundred percent convinced that this finding was the answer to all of my symptoms, but it was the first indication of anything I had been given.

As the years went by, I learned more about menopause, and discovered that any of those symptoms I had could have been attributed to perimenopause and menopause, but not one doctor ever mentioned menopause as a possibility. Not one.

Symptoms of perimenopause and menopause that we commonly hear about:
- Nightsweats
- Hot flashes
- Moodiness
- Insomnia
- Brain fog

But *these* symptoms could also be attributed to menopause:
- Dizziness
- Depression
- Digestive problems
- Increase in allergies
- Itchy Skin/rash
- Joint/muscle aches
- Vertigo
- Tingling sensations throughout the body
- Exhaustion

Night sweats were the worst for me. I honestly didn't know what was going on. I just thought, "What the hell? Why am I sweating at night? This is crazy." Some nights my sleep would be interrupted several times due to my sweat—and when I say "sweat," I mean I was drenched.

I sleep in a t-shirt and that's pretty much it. I would wake up with a soaking wet t-shirt, to the point that I had to get up in the middle of the night to change into a dry t-shirt. I would come back into the bed and see that the bed was wet from my sweat.

At that point, I couldn't change the sheets because my husband was asleep, so I would go get a towel and put it on top of the wet part of the sheet, so I could get back into a semi-dry bed. But then the issue was I was a little bit cold, because I was still wet from all the sweating, and it would all happen again several hours later.

The lack of sleep is no joke.

When you are trying to get up and go to work and you had your sleep interrupted two or three times overnight, life becomes very challenging. This is how I was operating most of that time. I was working on very little sleep, all while working and trying to get to the gym to train hard. It was exhausting.

The lack of sleep can mess with your hunger cues, and your hormones, and intensify cravings, which can lead to overeating or consuming foods you may not ordinarily consume. This is one of the reasons why losing weight in menopause can be tricky. It's not inherently the stress or lack of sleep itself that is the problem, but how we react to it. Becoming aware and understanding what is going on is crucial.

The lack of sleep, I think, was worse than when I had a newborn baby. When you bring home a newborn from the hospital, you're told that sleep is not going to be great, but you can "sleep when the baby sleeps," (although, as I mentioned, I personally never did that too much, anyway). But there's no similar pass with menopause. I look back on that time of my life, and I wonder how I survived. I had never realized what a big role sleep played in my life. Now, I value sleep more than I ever have. But during that time period, the lack of sleep I dealt with was about as bad as it got. But somehow, I managed to carry on.

I was surviving day to day, and for me, the one thing that kept my sanity in check was going to the gym. Once I signed on with my coach and started with his training plan, I became really focused, and my symptoms felt like they were dissipating a bit.

Strength training made a difference with my menopause symptoms. Everyone experiences menopause differently, so I can't say that what worked for me will work for you, but I will say that when I started getting into the gym and lifting heavy weight, and really pushing myself, that's when my symptoms started to ease up a bit. Did they completely go away? No, they didn't, but they certainly improved, and I attribute that to getting into a strength training routine.

I think one of the biggest myths that we believe when we reach this stage of life, is that it's over. By "it" I mean how our body looks. It's fate. It's a right of passage of sorts. It's inevitable. We will gain unwanted fat, and it will be impossible to get rid of it. That's what I always thought. The driver of this false belief is that we assume that as we age, our metabolism slows down. We assume that it slows down to the point of it being the sole cause for all of our fat gain.

I had assumed that my metabolism slowed way down. It was moving at a snail's pace. Everything I had heard confirmed the belief that as we get older, our metabolism slows way down. For years, I used that as my reasoning for why I was putting on weight, and why I couldn't lose fat. To me, this just made sense. It was the simple answer. It verified everything I thought to be true. I had gained fat, and that was why.

It's super easy to blame our weight gain on something outside of our control, so although I didn't like it, it was an easy way out. I looked at myself and I thought, this is as good as it's going to get.

I was convinced. I was convinced because I talked myself into thinking I had been doing everything right. I ate "healthy" and worked out a ton. What more does one have to do? I thought it was as good as it was going to get, but that couldn't be further from the truth.

What I wasn't doing was paying close attention to my nutrition. That would come back to haunt me in a big way.

I stayed in this phase of blaming menopause for quite some time. I wasn't tracking my food, or paying attention to any of that. I was eating "healthy," but I was still trying to blame my weight issues on something else besides myself.

It became increasingly frustrating as time went on. I thought my metabolism had slowed way down and was making it way more difficult (if not impossible) to lose weight. So I finally decided to get checked out. I went to see my doctor. That changed everything.

CHAPTER 10
IT'S GOTTA BE MY METABOLISM

I remember this day very, very well. I was 53 years old, I thought menopause was in full swing, and that I had lost all control. I remember standing in my bathroom one morning, crying while looking down at myself, saying, "What the hell has happened to me?"

My belly was sticking out, over fat thighs and hips that had gotten bigger.

How did I let this happen? The tears started. I was so upset. I felt like my body had betrayed me. I felt like I had gained significant weight overnight. It felt like I was out of control and I honestly didn't know what to do.

I was frustrated and I was angry. And I was also humiliated. I worked so hard in the gym and I was eating "clean" and healthy, and yet I continued to get bigger. What more does someone have to do?

It had to be my metabolism. There was no other explanation. I was convinced it was happening to me. It all made sense. The belly fat, the weight gain. My metabolism was as slow as a tortoise.

And to make matters even worse, I was a fitness professional. How the hell does a fitness professional not have her shit together—and end up like this? I was embarrassed and I was humiliated. I had to figure this out. I had to.

I think that morning was my "aha" moment that finally spurred on real change. It hit me like a ton of bricks that day. I'm not sure why that day was different than the previous days, but that morning, for some reason, was a turning point.

That morning, I came to the realization that it was time to figure it out. I made the appointment to go see my doctor. I wanted answers.

I was sitting in the waiting room of my doctor's office, and I was nervous (like I always am going to the doctor), but this time, I was a little bit excited, too, because I knew I was about to finally find the answers. I had planned out in my head exactly what was going to go down.

It was going to go something like this:

I figured I would start out by telling my doctor about my "unexplained" weight gain. I would give her some details about my background: I am a trained fitness professional. I workout at least six days a week, sometimes seven. I lift heavy weights. At that point, I figured she would get it, but I would continue on to describe how "clean" I was eating. I would list all the foods I ate, and all of the foods I would never allow to cross my lips. I figured she would be incredibly impressed with what I do, and would wholeheartedly agree with me that my weight gain is not due to lifestyle. That there has to be a medical reason for this.

I had convinced myself of this already, and I was certain my doctor would agree, and together we would get confirmation that I had some sort of thyroid or other hormone-related issue.

She would prescribe some medication and I would walk out that door, get my medication, start taking it, and poof! Everything will change. Finally. The relief I would feel would be enormous. That was how this was going to go down.

Well, I walked into the appointment and my doctor and I had a great conversation. But as we were talking, my emotions started coming to the surface. All of my frustration. All of my anger. All of my humiliation. All of those years of yo-yo dieting, restricting, losing weight, not able to sustain it, gaining weight again. Not being able to fit into my clothes. Over and over. All of it. It all started to boil over.

I started to cry. Right there in front of my doctor. I had been holding it in for years, and it was finally coming out.

She was kind, compassionate, and understood how devastated I was. She listened to everything I had to say, and came back with, "Let's order some blood work."

Those were the words I had been waiting to hear. Finally! We are moving forward. I pulled myself together and headed downstairs to the lab. I couldn't get there fast enough.

As I think back on that visit, my gut feeling is that she knew what was going on from the outset, but she listened, and validated everything I was feeling at the time, and went ahead and ordered the tests anyway.

I got the results fairly quickly, and went back to see my doctor. She said my blood work came back absolutely fine. There was nothing wrong with my metabolism at all, she said. As the words came out of her mouth, I felt like I had been punched in the gut. I was banking on having such a low metabolism that I was certain I would be put on medication.

Then, my doctor told me in a nice, but blunt way, "The problem is that you're eating too much."

Talk about "hard to hear." I just sat there, staring blankly. I didn't want to believe her, I didn't want to agree with her. Instantly, I had all kinds of thoughts go through my head:

"She's crazy."

"She's wrong."

"There must be a mistake."

"I eat healthy. What are you talking about?"

I couldn't (and didn't want to) wrap my head around

what she said.

You do something for so long, and you think you're doing it right. You think you're checking all the boxes. Seriously, you think you're doing everything the way you're supposed to be doing it, and you do it for many years...and then someone comes and tells you, "No, that's not how it is at all. You haven't been doing things right."

No, of course she didn't say in quite that way, but that's exactly what I heard: that I had screwed up, big time.

I'm a fitness professional. Holy shit, I really screwed up. A doctor just told me I was eating too much. The humiliation was real. The disappointment in myself was even worse. It was hard to hear in the moment, but I later thanked her for it. That conversation is what started the change for me.

But I wasn't ready to hear it that day. It took quite a while, actually, for me to accept what she said and to truly believe her.

I left the office in a terrible mood, but as the days went on, our conversation made me think. It got the wheels turning and, ultimately, gave me the push I needed to get off the hamster wheel I had been on for more than thirty years. It stopped my cycle of frustration of overly restricting what I was eating and not caring about portions, and going back and forth and back and forth, and then blaming something else for all of the weight gain and the yo-yoing.

As time went on, I became a little more focused on what I was eating and how much I was eating. I didn't do anything drastic. I just started to educate myself more in the area of nutrition. I became a consumer of educational content and research, started following highly respected people in the industry, and ultimately became more aware.

I have always said that awareness is one of the keys to success. We have to become consciously aware of what we put in our mouths every day, because if we don't, we will continue to underestimate the amount of calories we are eating, underestimate the portion sizes, and overestimate how consistent we are being.

Awareness is where change begins—and I was becoming truly aware for the first time.

I still wasn't tracking calories, because I still believed I didn't need to, but I was ultimately heading in that direction

As a coach, I still hear all the time how people think they gained weight because their metabolism has slowed down.

This part is super important: when we hit menopause, our metabolism does in fact slow down, but it doesn't slow down to the point that we can blame it for all of our weight gain, for all of our fat gain, or for us not making progress. It's not that significant.

So then, people say, "Okay, if it's not that, why does this happen to so many of us at this time of life?"

What Really Happens During Menopause?

Menopause is not some complex physiological phenomenon. It's actually not as complicated as we might think.

Now, I'm not saying that menopause doesn't play a role in any of this, because I think it does. During this time of life, things are going to be harder. Impossible? No. Harder? Admittedly, yes.

Symptoms of menopause will indeed make our lives, in general, a little tougher to get through. Hot flashes, night sweats, and hormonal changes are only the beginning. Our sleep can be affected, our hunger can be affected, and our mood can be affected, too, and all of these things can make it harder for us to lose weight. Plain and simple. Things are more challenging for us, but it doesn't make it impossible, like we might think it is.

Where people go wrong is when they blame everything on those physiological symptoms, instead of taking responsibility and making the necessary changes that will kick all of this in the ass.

That's what I want everyone to know: just because you're going through menopause and losing weight has become harder than it was before, doesn't mean you can't do it, or that you should give up trying.

Let's talk about this.

Over the course of twenty to thirty years (from as early as young adulthood) we tend to become less active. Little by little, day by day, over the course of time, our activity level drops. Maybe we used to chase our kids around when we were younger. Maybe we used to have a job that had us moving more when we were younger, but over time, our energy output has dropped. Our lives have changed. We get stressful jobs and are working a lot, our kids have schedules, and we become less active. And because this happens slowly, over the course of so many years, we don't even notice it.

Our energy output has decreased, and as a result, we are losing muscle mass as we go along. We become way less efficient calorie burners overall.

Plus, our nutrition gets lost along the way. We eat on the run, more often than not. We are getting meals on the road, enroute to our kids' practices. We don't have the time to plan out meals at home. We just don't have a handle on our nutrition like we think we do.

And we want to still be able to eat like we did when we were in our twenties. And we often still try to.

Everyone else's needs are coming before ours. This is a typical pattern, starting in your thirties (maybe even earlier) and continues on over the course of twenty to thirty years.

You combine all of that with being less active, and you have the perfect storm for weight gain.

Mother Nature was getting ready to mess with us anyway, but we've helped her right along for years. We've been less active, we haven't paid that much attention to our nutrition, and with Mother Nature's help, boom, here we are.

It's easy to turn around and say, "Yeah, it's all menopause." But it's not all menopause.

Does our metabolism actually slow down? Yes, to a point, and if you have not been exercising or strength training along the way, you will lose some muscle mass. And when you lose muscle mass, your metabolic rate goes down, which means you don't burn calories at the same rate you used to.

I think all of us, at some point, think we can still do things like we did when we were in our twenties. Everything from running, to lifting heavy things, to eating. We can still do it all. And in some cases, we do.

Have you ever said something to the effect of, "I used to be able to eat like this when I was younger, but not anymore?"

The reason that statement holds true is because you aren't moving as much as you used to. You haven't been working out as much (or at all). It's not because of menopause itself, but because your habits, over the course of many years, have changed.

The metabolic drop that has happened is more from your habits, than it is from your age.

Let me repeat that: The metabolic drop that has happened is more from your habits than it is from your age.

Combine that with not paying too much attention to our nutrition, and hello, weight gain.

One thing I want to point out here is that some of you could very well be diagnosed with a metabolic problem or other physiological condition that can make fat loss much more challenging. If you fall into that category, work with your doctor on what treatments are available for you. When metabolism issues are treated, it makes losing weight a bit easier—but make no mistake the science of weight loss still holds true. You need to consume less calories than your body needs. The challenge can become finding what that number is. The number may be lower, and it may be more challenging, but it is still possible to do whether you have a diagnosed condition or not.

So, you have a choice here.

It may be harder to lose weight in menopause. In fact, I think for most of us it is.

What are you going to do about it?

Are you going to say that it's too hard, give up, and not do anything about it, or are you going to say yes, it's hard, and keep moving forward anyway?

That's the question you need to ask yourself. And when you're ready to tackle it, that's when you're going to start making progress.

It takes owning up to what's been going on, it takes owning up to what you have to do, it takes consistency, and it takes patience. Keep after it.

It's never too late for you to change. It might be harder, but it's never too late. That is the ultimate difference. When it gets tougher, you have to buckle down and get tougher, too.

The seed my doctor planted in my head that day grew. I finally started zeroing in on my nutrition, more specifically than just eating healthy. Between that and the coach I was about to hire, my life was about to change in a great way.

CHAPTER 11
AND THE CHANGE BEGAN

As I let the words of my doctor sink in, I started to fully realize that if I wanted to lose weight, I needed to start making some changes. I still wasn't sold on the idea of counting or tracking calories just yet, but I was becoming more aware of what I was consuming throughout the course of the day, and awareness is where it all has to begin.

I was cutting back on the handfuls of almonds and bites of trail mix a bit. I was making my lattes with skim instead of whole milk. Baby steps like that.

I also started to focus more on protein. How was I going to get more protein in my diet?

While taking these baby steps nutritionally, I continued to strength train, and my love for it grew even stronger. I loved the challenge it brought, I loved the strength I was gaining, and I loved the confidence I felt.

As a result, I started looking into competing in a powerlifting meet. Doing something like that was way out of my comfort zone, but it seemed like a great goal to work toward. Everyone I have ever spoken to about powerlifting has had nothing but amazing things to say about the meet, about how supportive the competitors are and the powerlifting community is in general, and just what a great experience it was.

I was excited.

I spoke with a few people who did competitions, and they all told me they had coaches who trained them in preparation for the meet. Some coaches actually went to the meet with them and became their "handler" — the person who helped get the competitor warmed up, made sure the competitor was where they needed to be on time, and their main support system for the meet.

So, I needed a coach.

I had worked with many trainers throughout the years, but none of them were powerlifters and I didn't have any local connections, so I began to think about hiring an online coach. I had never worked with an online coach before, and I didn't one hundred percent understand how it all worked, but I did know that I was highly motivated, and if I truly wanted to compete in a powerlifting meet, I was going to need a coach who understood the process. They needed to be okay with how little I knew about powerlifting, and understand how intimidating this would be for me. The thought of all this made me so nervous I thought I would throw up, but it also made me so excited

I couldn't sit still.

One of my trainer colleagues whom I had met online (she was from the midwest), had competed in a powerlifting meet, and she told me all about it. This continued my excitement, so I asked her who she recommended me to hire as my powerlifting coach. She said, without hesitation, to hire the coach she had: a man named Jordan Syatt.

Well, I already knew who Jordan Syatt was, as I was already on his email list and got regular emails from him. I had discovered his content online and loved his vibe. He definitely knew his stuff, that was obvious—he was a world record powerlifter. After watching some of his videos and reading a ton of his articles, I got a good gut feeling about hiring him. I had a feeling he was going to be the right coach for me.

And my gut about people has never really been wrong.

I filled out the coaching inquiry form on his website. I let it sit for hours without sending it. I was so nervous. I desperately wanted to do this, but I almost did not hit "send." I started to question myself, my abilities, finances, everything. But really, what I was doing was making excuses.

So I hit send.

I was anxious. I had worked with trainers before, but none of his caliber, and certainly no one online. I had no clue if Jordan would even want to work with someone like me, but I knew I had to give this a try. I was simultaneously curious, terrified, and excited.

Jordan responded quickly and we set up a consult call. Jordan was living in Israel at the time, and I remember being thankful that he did the time zone math to set up the call, because I screw up simple time zone calculations all the time. Little did I know, that consult call would change my life.

Jordan says he remembers that call well. I can't say the same. I was so nervous my stomach was in knots and my memory wasn't functioning well. I can't remember exactly what I said, but I remember exactly how I felt.

During our conversation, I remember thinking, "This guy gets it." Something just felt right, like he understood my drive and my desire to get strong. Although I was still nervous, I felt comfortable. My gut told me this guy would be a great fit for me, and my gut was right.

He was confident that I was a good fit for his coaching as well. When I hung up the phone, I had a boost of confidence like I hadn't felt in a long time. I couldn't wait to get started.

One of the first things Jordan did was send me a form to fill out about goals, equipment availability, and questions about my overall knowledge base. He also asked me to film myself doing a couple basic lifts so he could see me move and give me some critique on my technique.

I loved taking on the role of "good student" again. I am a rule follower, a pleaser, and—though I am definitely not the most talented person—I will work harder than most. I wanted my coach's first impression of me to be a strong one, so I took great care in videoing my deadlift and squat to send him.

He said he loved my videos and mentioned some things we would work on, but overall he thought my technique was great. I was super happy. We were on our way.

I received my first training program soon thereafter. I took one look at it and thought, "This is it?" I was working out six or seven days a week, with lots and lots of sets and reps, sometimes even doing two-a-days. I was expecting pages of exercises with lots of volume. But my first program with Jordan?

Four Days a week. One lower body day, one upper body day, another lower body day, and another upper body day, with only a handful of exercises on each day.

Each workout day had maybe five exercises at most, with only three sets of each. I thought I was missing an entire page, or maybe two! It didn't seem like much on paper. Then I started wondering what I was supposed to do on the other three days of the week. There were no instructions, no separate pages for those days. So clearly, something was missing.

So I asked him, "What should I do on the off days? I don't see anything for that."

His response?

"Rest."

Wait, what? REST?
No, I don't want to rest. I want to work.

I was coming from the "more is better" camp. As I

mentioned back in Chapter 6, I worked out a lot, and I thought the more I worked out, the better.

My new program couldn't possibly have enough exercises and volume. It was way less than I was used to, and I started to panic a bit. I thought that if I did not workout as much as I had been, I would lose progress and get fat. I couldn't ever remember taking a purposeful rest day. Rest was for the weak—or so I thought.

After my initial panic, I decided I was going to have to trust this process, trust Jordan, and follow the rules. I knew that when you do follow instructions, usually good things will happen. As scared as I was, I trusted Jordan, and was going to give it a go.

The first scheduled rest day was hell. Pure hell. I felt fidgety, very uncomfortable, and anxious. I communicated this to Jordan.

I am sure there was a lot of eye rolling on his end. I bet he was thinking, "Oh boy, here we go. She's one of 'those people'.'"

Probably just to shut me up, Jordan told me, "OK, OK, you can go to the gym. Go sit on a bike and do some low-intensity, steady state cardio—but don't let your heart rate get up."

Perfect! I got my permission to get to the gym, so off I went. I hopped on a spin bike, and started to pedal. About five minutes in, while trying to keep my heart rate down, I was still antsy. I wanted to push, but I was a rule follower. I tried listening to music, or watching one of the many TVs in front of me, but I was struggling to keep my sanity at this low pace.

I was miserable.

I learned one very valuable lesson that day: low-intensity, steady state cardio was not my thing (at least for now). I guess that's why, up until that point, I did not enjoy walking. When I would go for a walk, I couldn't just walk. I had to walk with purpose. Get the heart rate up. Work. At that time, I wasn't able to just walk and enjoy it. Several years later, that would change, but I'm getting ahead of myself.

After my session, I messaged Jordan and told him I almost lost my mind, and that moving forward, I would follow the rules to the "T." I am certain Jordan got a big kick out of that. Four Days of training. Three Rest days. Here I come.

My first month's program came around the same time the National Weather Service was predicting a blizzard would hit in my area.

The Washington D.C. area does not "do" snow well. Two inches is a disaster, never mind a blizzard. The slightest bit of snow and everything shuts down, the roads are horrible, and everyone runs out to grab eggs, milk, and toilet paper from the grocery store, so the prospect of a legitimate blizzard meant a potential shut down for several days. And when you live in a cul-de-sac on a dead end street, seeing a snow plow come through is a rare sight.

Being the rule follower that I am, I was still determined not to miss any of my workouts. Blizzard or not. I started to look at my program and see what I could do from home, in case I got snowed in.

I have a home gym downstairs in the extra room that was supposed to be a "family room," with a TV, some comfy chairs, and so on. There is a sliding glass door that opens up to three stone steps away from the pool deck. It's a pretty nice set up. Only one problem: before I took up building a home gym, no one used the room at all.

Since no one ever used that room, I took it upon myself to change it up a little. Out went the furniture and in came a squat rack, a bunch of plates, a DB rack, a bench, and some other odds and ends. This space became my home gym, and eventually the space where I trained people in person. It was actually set up primarily to train others. I personally preferred to get out of the house and go to the gym for my own workouts. To me, home was home. A place to unwind and relax, not lift as much weight as I could.

But with a blizzard coming, my home gym was going to come in handy. I could get through my entire program, except one critical exercise: Chin ups.

Chin ups were a goal of mine and became a main focus for me. In my opinion, they represent the ultimate in strength. They are an exercise that many women struggle with, and I was one of those women. I had never done a chin up. Not one. Ever. I was that kid in elementary school who hated those PE tests that included the flex arm hang. I couldn't hold a flex arm hang for more than one second.

Basically, I couldn't hold it at all.

I was always embarrassed by that. Other kids would laugh, and I would laugh along with them to try and save face. In my memory, everyone—literally everyone—could do the flex arm hang but me. While I am not one hundred percent certain of how accurate my memory is regarding that experience, the sense of embarrassment and humiliation was real.

Chin ups were the one exercise I didn't want to skip in my new program. The issue wasn't that I didn't have a chin up bar, because I did. The issue was that it was located outside, and we were expecting blizzard conditions. Granted, it was mounted on the side of my deck and was partially covered, but we were expecting two feet of snow with heavy winds, with temperatures and wind chill hovering in the low teens.

It was not the best time to be outside, to say the least.

I think some people may have just said, screw it. And for good reason, really. We were about to get hammered with snow and high winds. No one would want to go outside in those conditions. Especially to do chin ups.

No one...except me.

As I said earlier, I was a rule follower. The day the blizzard came, I had chin ups on my program—and dammit, I was going to do chin ups. Yup, I was going to do chin ups outside in the blizzard, because that was on my program. I didn't want Jordan to think I was one of those clients who has a litany of excuses as to why they can't do something. I knew he wouldn't think that, but he was from Boston, and snow doesn't phase those folks up there, so I wasn't going to let snow phase me.

So, out in the blizzard I went. I made my son go with me so he could film it. I wanted to show Jordan that there was no way in hell I was going to let a blizzard stop me from working to get my first chin up. I was doing chin ups with an assist band at the time, so I had my band with me as outside I went.

I was bundled up in my Batman tights, lots of layers, hat, gloves, everything. I anchored my band, and put in my assisted chin ups outside with temps in the teens, snow blowing everywhere, and freezing my butt off.

I was driven. I didn't want my coach to think anything else but, "She's determined." Jordan and I talk about that video all the time. It definitely made an impression on him, and it really set the level of expectation I set for myself—which was something I needed.

As we continued working together, I became a believer in the fact that I didn't have to work out six or seven days a week any more in order to make progress. I finally started to see the benefits in taking real, legitimate rest days. I felt better, I was sleeping better, and my workouts were much better. They were much more effective, and I was starting to see it.

Why was it different this time? I had had coaches before, and had worked hard previously. I think this time, with a new coach, a new perspective, a new way of training, and having someone who I finally felt genuinely cared about me and my progress, I started to feel different. I loved getting his feedback, I loved learning more and more about technique, and I loved the feeling of getting stronger and stronger. Surrounding yourself with the right people can make all the difference. And it most certainly did for me.

When I started working with Jordan, he offered nutrition coaching as well, but I didn't do any official nutrition coaching with him for a couple misguided reasons:

1. I had started losing some fat before I started to work with him, as indicated by how my clothes started to fit differently. Although I still wasn't tracking what I was eating, I was becoming more aware of how much I was eating and made small adjustments along the way. Nothing drastic by any stretch of the imagination, but it was working (a little), and I mistakenly thought that meant I had it all figured out.

2. I immediately believed my short term fat loss would automatically translate into long term success.

But I had no real plan. I was eating a little less, but I was still kind of winging it.

My relationship with food was still the same: there were "good" foods and there were "bad" foods, and I still struggled with allowing myself to have certain foods without feeling guilty or anxious.

Since I wasn't officially doing nutrition coaching with Jordan, we didn't talk too much about nutrition at the beginning. Things were primarily focused around training. But just because I wasn't getting any official nutrition coaching from Jordan doesn't mean I wasn't paying attention.

Remember, I was a good student. I read every article Jordan wrote, I watched every video he made, and I started to put some things into practice. I was slowly learning the basics about nutrition for fat loss, and was beginning to see how it could all come together.

I also took another big step: I joined Jordan's Inner Circle. The Inner Circle is an online fitness community with monthly workouts, monthly nutrition guidelines, a members' portal that contains a wealth of valuable content, and a members-only Facebook community. I was eager to learn as much as I could from this guy, so I wanted to be exposed to all of his content.

My workouts were progressing nicely. The strength gains were starting to appear. And nutrition? I was making tremendous strides there as well. My strength was increasing, and I was starting to see some muscle definition, too, which was a huge motivator for me. This was a big reason for my eventual switch in focus from powerlifting to more aesthetic-based goals and building muscle.

During this time, I was following the program Jordan wrote for me to the "T." I also started following the nutrition guidelines that were in the monthly Inner Circle Editions. These nutrition guidelines consisted of how to calculate your daily calorie goal, and how to calculate your daily protein goal for fat loss.

I calculated both, and started tracking. I had never consistently tracked before. I decided I didn't want to use an app to help track, and I still don't to this day. This is a total old school approach, but it works for me. It ultimately doesn't matter how you track; what's important is finding what works for you. Most people are stunned that I don't use an app, and many even laugh at my age showing through. This is when I most feel like the "Get Off My Lawn" type of old person. Everyone is using an app for everything.

Everyone but me.

I know, I know. They do so much. They can calculate, they can scan, they might even be able to cook your dinner—who knows? I just knew that using an app was going to be way more complicated for me than it should be. I didn't want to add yet another piece of technology that I had to deal with on my to-do list, so I took a different route than just about everybody.

I have come a long way with technology, but there are just some things I would rather do on paper.

So, I started tracking my calories on paper. I wrote everything in my notebook by hand: the food, how much, the calories, and the protein (if applicable). I continued this way for quite some time, and it worked well, but eventually I moved to a simple spreadsheet on my computer.

I switched to a spreadsheet because it would do the math for me, and any of the math teachers I had at any point in my education would wholeheartedly agree: this was a good move. Math was never my forte. In fact, I have jokingly said that the day percentages were taught in whatever grade that was, I must have been absent, because I have struggled with percentages ever since.

Tracking was eye opening. It blatantly pointed out a few different things:

- It was not as hard as I thought
- We as humans suck at estimating calories and portion sizes. My estimation was incredibly far off.

I find it fascinating how bad we humans are at estimating calories. We all suck at it. What we think is four ounces is actually six. What we think is six hundred calories is actually nine hundred. Weighing your food along with tracking is the best thing you can do to truly learn accurate portion sizes. It's eye opening. Portion sizes are where most people go wrong, including me. Especially me.

Tracking calories is something that I encourage everyone to do at some point. It's not something you have to do forever, like I used to think, but if you do it for an extended period of time, what you learn will be extremely valuable. The education you will get about calories, portion sizes and protein grams will take you through your entire life. It will make whatever journey you are on—be it fat loss, muscle building, or even maintaining—much, much smoother.

Tracking will help you become empowered and knowledgeable. I will cover details about tracking and exactly how to set it all up in Chapter 16.

Originally, I hired my coach for powerlifting, but as I soon found out, I needed him for way more than that. I thought I knew the rest and could figure it all out on my own, but what I learned was that even coaches need coaches. And when you find the right one, things start to change. As I kept learning, putting things into practice, and trusting his process, I started seeing results. This motivated me to learn even more and to keep working hard.

Deep down, I thought I would always be a Yo-Yo dieter, but with my new coach on board, my newfound approach to training, and finally getting a handle on my nutrition, I was about to prove myself wrong.

VERY wrong.

CHAPTER 12
OVERCOMING FEAR AND THE SCALE

As my training and newfound nutrition focus continued, I started to see big changes. My strength was increasing, and my clothes started to fit differently. They felt looser, which is a sign that change is happening. But there was one change in particular that started to show its face more and more.

Confidence.

I had always felt fairly confident in the gym, but even I had some moments of intimidation, nerves, and self-consciousness.

I think we all go through periods of feeling self-conscious in the gym.

We think everyone is looking at us, judging us, and making fun of us.

We think we are the focus of everyone's thoughts as we enter the gym.

We think they're all thinking, Who is that person?

What is she doing here? She has no clue what she is doing.

But that's not reality. There is probably not one single person in the gym who is thinking any of those things.

I have worked with many people over the years who have told me they prefer to workout at home not because of convenience, but because they are too intimidated to go to the gym. They are afraid of not performing exercises correctly, they are afraid of people making fun of them, and they are afraid of other people judging them. They also say they are intimidated by people who can lift significant amounts of weight when they might just be starting out.

One thing I have learned from being in a gym is that those big burly guys who lift a ton and who look intimidating aren't intimidating at all. Most are super nice people, who would actually applaud the efforts of someone coming in and being fairly new to the lifting environment. And, more often than not, they are willing to help you.

One of the main reasons for "gym intimidation" is not having a plan when you arrive. You walk into the gym not having a clue as to what you are going to work on. You can't remember a single exercise you saw online. You can't remember sets, reps, or anything. So one of two scenarios usually happens:

Scenario 1

You walk into the gym, and start to meander around the free weight section, not knowing what to do. Then, head over to the cable station. You proceed to do a handful of lat pull downs and then a handful of bicep curls. The weight is pretty light, the cable is moving freely, and there is not a lot of intensity. You repeat those two exercises. Then you meander around the gym again, and then leave. I have seen that exact scenario happen in my own gym more times than I can count. It becomes blatantly obvious that the person either forgot what they were intending to do or, more likely, they didn't have a plan at all. They just did what they knew, and left.

Scenario 2

You walk into the gym with every intention of going into the free weight section of the gym. You had reviewed a few exercises from social media prior, but as you get closer to the free weight section, you see all the people there who appear to know exactly what they are doing. You begin to freeze up. You start getting scared. What if people start looking at me? What if they are judging me? You then do an about-face and hop on the elliptical, where you stay for at least thirty minutes.

Deep down inside, I believe most people want to go to the weight section of the gym. They want to get stronger and build some muscle, but fear takes over. When I talk to people about this, we have to have a bit of a reality check. They are allowing random people in the gym to keep them from reaching their goals. Think about that. They are allowing people they don't even know, people who have never spoken a single word to them before, dictate their own actions.

When you say that out loud, it sounds crazy, right? But this happens all the time.

One of the main reasons people don't want to go to the gym or are intimidated to go to the gym is because they don't know what to do. They don't have a program. They don't have a plan, so they end up wandering around the gym (like Scenario 1), trying to remember the exercises they saw on social media. And when they can't remember any of them, they end up doing a few bicep curls (it's always bicep curls), or head on over to the cardio machines (like Scenario 2) and watch TV while on the elliptical.

There is a constant fear of looking stupid, of having people judge them and even laugh at them. Going to the gym becomes more stressful, when it is supposed to be stress relieving. It becomes an unpleasant experience, and so, many people end up not going at all. It's just easier going for a walk instead.

This is why having a plan is so crucial.

Here are my three steps for getting over gym intimidation

1. **Have a workout plan.** Know what you are going to do: the exact exercises, sets, and reps. Write everything down and predetermine what you will do. If you don't know what to do, you could get a program online, or get a coach to write one that is tailored just for you.

2. **Review it before you go.** Look it over. Even have access to video demos of the exercises that you can refer to while in the gym, in case your mind draws a big fat blank (which happens all the time).

3. **Stick with your program.** If you start to feel uncomfortable, keep going. If you start feeling anxious, keep thinking about how you will feel at the end. The feeling of accomplishment. The feeling of confidence. The feeling of, "I did it." Thinking about how you will feel afterward is super important.

Most of all, remember that this will take practice. It won't be a switch that you flip from off to on. It will be gradual. Each time you go, each time you fight through the discomfort, and each time you complete your program, you will feel stronger, more confident, and—before you know it—like you own the place.

The confidence that I started feeling was getting bigger and bigger as time went on. I felt completely comfortable in the gym. I started making "gym friends." these people were always there when I was. These familiar faces were people I spoke to, but I had no idea what their names were. They became my new circle of nameless friends.

I started to feel like I owned the place.

As I continued along with my training program and following along the Inner Circle nutrition guidelines, changes were happening. My strength was increasing rapidly and I was starting to notice changes in my body. My clothes were fitting even better than before, and I was starting to see my muscles come through. I was sure I was losing some weight.

But the kicker?

I didn't own a bathroom scale.

What?

Yep. I didn't own a scale.

My parents had a scale in my house growing up, but I never personally owned one until recently. I did step on a scale though—every time I went to the doctor. That was it.

Every doctor's visit was riddled with anxiety, not because of what I was actually there for, but because I was going to have to step on their scale. Just that made me nervous and anxious.

My heart would pound in my chest in the waiting room. The nurse would have me step on the Physician beam scale, and she would slide those bars from left to right until the balance arm was centered. When the nurse would start to move that big bar, I remember wanting to scream, "STOP!" The end result was either going to make me upset because it was more than I wanted, or it was going to make me happy because it was less than I expected. All these emotions, just because of a number. For years and years, this would be the case. I was allowing a number to completely dictate how I felt about myself. I attached so much emotion and self-worth to a stupid number. The scale had so much power over me for so many years, and I didn't even realize it at the time.

The fear of the scale was owning me. I was afraid of it, and I was tired of feeling that way, so a few years ago I decided it was time and finally bought myself a bathroom scale.

Truthfully, I was afraid of it because I didn't understand it, and it was time to fix that.

So let's talk about scale fluctuations.

The scale fluctuates daily. Sometimes a lot, sometimes a little. There are so many things that can affect scale fluctuation, but the only thing I was thinking at the time was that if it went up, that was bad. If it went down, that was good

When you step on the scale, it is measuring the weight of your bones, your tendons, your muscle, your organs, your water, your ligaments, and your fat. It weighs everything, not just fat—but when we see the scale fluctuate on a daily basis, we assume it's all about gaining and losing fat. If the scale goes up a pound overnight, you automatically think you've gained a pound of fat, but daily fluctuations on the scale are mostly related to water. You are either holding on to water, or you have let go of some water.

If you were to step on a scale multiple times a day (please do not do this!), you would see fluctuations all day long, mostly because of water (along with having more or less content in your stomach).

When you retain water, you are going to weigh more. So why do you retain water?

Maybe you had more carbs the day before. When you eat more carbs, you will retain water. The glycogen in carbs also contains water. Water retention when eating carbs is normal. If you ate more carbs than normal, you may be retaining more water than normal.

Maybe you ate more salty foods than normal. Salty foods will make you retain water, as well. For me, Chinese food is a biggie. Every time I eat Chinese food, regardless of the quantity, I can expect at least a pound increase on the scale the next morning.

Maybe you lifted heavy weights the day before. When you lift heavy weights, you break down your muscle fibers and they repair themselves. That's how you build strength. During the repair process, your muscles will hold onto water as well.

Other reasons the scale may fluctuate?

Maybe you need to poop. Seriously. Do your bathroom thing first, then step on the scale. And if you want to try a fun experiment, try this:

Step on the scale before you pee. Then go pee. Then step on the scale and see the difference.

Make sure you are weighing at the same time every day.

Make sure you are using the same scale every time you weigh in.

Track your daily scale weight, but only compare the numbers monthly. This is super important to understand. You can't compare Monday's scale weight to Tuesday's scale weight. Day-to-day numbers are meaningless, really, especially for the first thirty days. What is going to paint a way more accurate picture is comparing the number from the first of the month to the first of next month and start looking for trends.

If you were to graph thirty days of scale weight, you would probably see something like this:

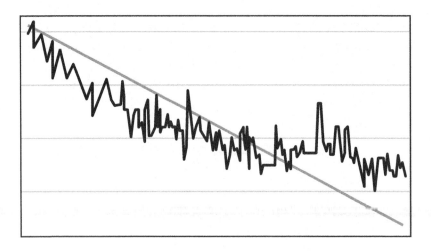

There are a lot of peaks and valleys in this chart, but if you were to draw a straight line from the beginning to the very end, the trend is down. It may look more like a heart rate monitor than a weight loss pattern, but this is a very typical pattern. However, most people quit when they see the day-to-day weight spikes. They panic, and think their nutrition plan is not working, but if you look at that graph, you will see what will happen if they just wait it out and keep going after a spike: they will see a dip, or what is better known as a "woosh." A woosh is you releasing that water you were retaining. Sometimes wooshes happen within a day or two, and sometimes it takes longer, but if you just keep going, things keep moving,

While the scale can be massively frustrating, the more you understand what is really going on, the better you will become at taking the emotion out of that number. Soon, you will be able to see the data for what it is: data.

Scale data is super helpful in analyzing your weight loss (or muscle gain) progress, but it shouldn't be the only method of assessing your progress.

Scale data in combination with other signs of progress (such as how you are feeling, how your clothes fit, your measurements, how you are sleeping, and how your strength has increased) gives you a much more complete picture of how you are progressing. The scale is not the only data point to consider.

So, I finally decided to get a scale and start weighing myself every single day. I wasn't specifically trying to lose fat at this point; I was just trying to get used to weighing myself and watching what the scale did, day in and day out. Learning was my goal.

I wanted to experience feeling "perfect" with my training and nutrition, yet still seeing the scale spike. I wanted to experience the feeling of seeing the scale dip down for no apparent reason. I wanted to experience it all. I wanted to learn how my own weight fluctuates day in and day out, and what it really means and doesn't mean.

Not only was I going to weigh myself, but I decided to post it on social media as well, to help others watch me go through the normal fluctuations that we all go through. Talk about fear! Talk about uncomfortable. I was very uncomfortable, but I also knew that doing this was not only going to help me learn more about my own body, but it was hopefully going to help others who might be feeling the same fear I was feeling: the fear of seeing the scale go up.

The very first day I weighed in, I was incredibly nervous. The anxiety was bad. And when I posted my weight on social media for the first time, I almost threw up.

But I posted it. I talked a lot on social media and on podcasts about how uncomfortable this made me, how I was conquering my own fear, and how I wanted to help others to do the same. I think that really helped me a lot. I also got a ton of messages of support from people who could completely relate to how I was feeling.

And so I did it. Every day, for almost three months, I posted my weight. I had weight spikes and dips along the way, which all evened themselves out. It was a fascinating process to watch unfold.

I cannot begin to say how much I learned from that experience. I logically knew about scale fluctuations, but could never think of them beyond the emotion, whether it was good or bad. Seeing the daily fluctuations became fascinating as time went on. I was getting pretty good at predicting what my weight would be as I learned what affected it. As I kept going, the powerful grip the scale had on me started to loosen up and eventually let go.

I conquered that fear by facing it head on. That's how you have to conquer any fear: By facing it and dealing with it. Not avoiding it. If you avoid it, you will always be afraid. It will own you. If you face it head on, you will eventually win.

Do you have similar fears about the scale? My suggestion is to step on the scale daily. Not weekly or monthly, but daily, so you can see the random spikes, wooshes, and trends over time. Now, they are a normal part of life. You can experience a random spike on the scale even when you feel you have been perfect with diet and exercise and not freak out, because you know you are retaining more water. Then, you can also experience a "woosh" as your body lets go of the water. If you only weigh-in once a week, you will miss a lot.

Removing emotions from the scale takes time, consistent practice, and maybe even a few conversations with yourself. You may need to remind yourself of the differences between day to day fluctuations versus trends over time.

I would be completely lying if I said I don't get a small kick in the gut when I see the scale go up, but the difference now is that the feeling only lasts briefly, and I don't allow that feeling to dictate what I do next.

It's a massive win, and a massive boost in self-efficacy and self-confidence.

Weighing myself was the first of many fears I would begin to conquer.

CHAPTER 13
A BUSINESS IS BORN

Building a training business on my own wasn't something I considered right away. I sort of assumed I would get a part-time job at a gym, train people there, and that would be it. And that's what happened. For a while.

My first personal training job was a part-time gig while I was still a school counselor. I was super excited and nervous to give this a shot. I knew I had a lot to learn, but I also felt prepared from my teaching and counseling background.

I was one of three trainers at this very small gym and I was well received. I was very different from the other two trainers who were there. For starters, I was the only female, and I was also about twice their age (or somewhere thereabouts). The fact that I was older seemed to be very appealing to the clientele. The feedback I got was that people were happy to see someone who was closer to their age teaching people how to lift, because they felt like they could relate to me.

This was my first indication of how strong the middle-aged market actually was. There are a lot of middle-agers out there, and most want to take better care of themselves than their parents did. They want to live longer lives and be able to get strong, move well, and lose some fat—and they want to learn how to do it by someone they can relate to.

As well as my age, my teaching and counseling background made me stand out. One day, one of the other trainers was watching me teach someone a lift. He watched me break it down for the client, and get the client to perform the exercise correctly. This trainer approached me later and said he was so impressed by how I taught. And I just thought, that's what a teacher does. It was normal for me. It's what I knew how to do well.

My teaching background was (and still is) a definite strength for me as a coach.

Retirement from the school system was looming. I was excited, but terrified all at the same time. Education was all I had known, from the days of being a student myself and the days of my first teaching job. I had never been out of the education system or the education calendar. Being an educator was my identity. It was who I was.

My biggest concern about retiring was losing that identity. I never realized just how important my identity as an educator and counselor meant to me until I was about to lose it. I knew education. I knew it really well.

The thought of not being around it or a part of it was sad to me. It was like leaving your very best friend after working with them for thirty-three years—which is how long I had been in education. Thirty-three years is a long time for anything. It was the majority of my life, so leaving the comfort of what I knew so well was going to be hard. I have often said change is hard, but I truly think change gets more difficult the older you get.

That said, there was going to be a familiar thread. I was leaving the school, but I was still an educator. I became a counselor to help people. That's what I loved, to be able to sit down with kids and their families, and help them work through school and academic issues, whether it was grades, or the family needing assistance outside of school. I loved listening, speaking, and developing relationships with all of them. And I still got to do that part at the gym.

Leaving what I have known for so long wasn't going to be easy, but with my part-time training job, I was starting to see another door opening up as one was closing.

With Retirement on the horizon, I began training several of the staff members after school for free. The middle school I worked at had a legitimate weight room. The machines in there were smaller and more geared to younger kids' height, but there was a full dumbbell rack up to fifty pounds, as well as a few spin bikes. I used to use that weight room all the time after school to get a quick workout in. It was extremely convenient, very private (not used much by the staff), and had enough equipment for me to do what I wanted to do.

Some of the staff members would ask, now and then, if they could come down to the weight room and work out with me. Over time I gained a couple of regulars, and what ended up happening was me walking them through a workout session, then I got my own workout in afterward. I never charged a cent at the beginning. My reason for not charging was that I honestly didn't know what to charge, and I really wanted the experience of training people. I was having fun, they were having fun, and the interest started to grow. While some business "gurus" would look at that and say, "don't devalue your service," I looked at it as an opportunity to help people, get experience, and build interest, which is exactly what happened.

After I retired, I continued with training sessions at the school as the interest was still there and growing. I created a small-group training format, where I would work with a few people at a time. It still felt like personal training, but there were a few people instead of just one. What started with a few people, soon grew into fifteen.

Unbeknownst to me, this was the official start to Susan Niebergall Fitness.

I really liked that I was in charge. And I loved working with my former colleagues. My dream of training people had evolved from a very part-time side gig at a gym to the potential of training people out on my own. It was a scary but exciting proposition.

I wanted to make my in-person training business "official," so I had to have someone walk me through the LLC process. I didn't even know what LLC was, but a friend who owned her own business told me I needed to look into it. The business world was a scary, scary place for me. So much of the language used I didn't even understand. You might as well have been speaking a foreign language.

I had never taken a business class in my life, so I was the ultimate rookie. Luckily, I had a wonderful neighbor who had her own business teaching yoga out of her house. She, along with some other friends, walked me through the process and helped translate documents for me.

I eventually got through it all, and Susan Niebergall Fitness was official.

As the group in the middle school grew, I decided to leave the gym I had been working at so I could focus more on building my own in-person training business. I started charging minimal monthly fees, and started paying the county to officially rent some space. I held two sessions, twice a week. Coming from the education world myself, I knew that teachers sometimes had students staying after school for extra help, so I developed a teacher-friendly schedule with that in mind.

I provided two group coaching sessions: one right after school, and one after the schools' activity period, so the teachers could come to whichever fit their schedule the best. If they had students stay after school with them, they could see their students and then come to workout, or if they didn't have any students staying with them, they could come directly after school.

Teachers were hungry for a program like this. I think they are at most any school. Finding a program that was something they could afford (teachers don't get paid a lot anywhere) and was convenient were the two most important factors when trying to create something that worked for them, and this program did both.

I brought in a good friend of mine, Lars Kroner, to help coach them with me so we could accommodate more people as the interest grew. He and I were always on the same page, and he was the perfect fit with this crew.

We built quite a program there. I added some of my own equipment to the middle school gym over time, so we not only had access to dumbbells and some machines, but now some bars, plates, a squat rack, some KBs, and other assorted odds and ends as well. We had a total of four sessions per week. They deadlifted, they squatted, they pressed, they pulled, and they got strong.

We did fun things like having a Personal Record Day, where everyone would test how much weight they could move on a specific lift (usually a deadlift). Watching them cheer each other on and watching their faces as they used great technique to lift more weight off the floor than they ever imagined possible was priceless.

We gave out nutrition guidelines that included information on how to set their calories and protein for fat loss. Sometimes we would even run a nutrition challenge. The person who hit their calorie and protein targets the most in a given time period would win. Usually the prize was something like a big jug of protein.

One of the most interesting things about our group was that we had all ages represented. We had people in their twenties, someone almost seventy, and every age in between, and everyone was able to access every exercise. Sometimes, as people get older, they can be intimidated to use equipment like a barbell—but age was not a limiting factor here. Of course, everyone lifted the appropriate amount of weight for them, but the actual exercises were for everyone. This hammers home how age is not a barrier for strength training. Anyone can (and should) strength train, and everyone, regardless of how old they are, can benefit from it.

This group program, along with training individuals one to one at my home studio, was Susan Niebergall Fitness.

However, as most trainers who set out to help people discover, you are inherently limited with the number of people you can help in person. It's really just a time-to-person ratio. Group training can help this a little, but there are only so many hours of the day.

I wanted to expand my reach and help more people. The next step was going to take me so far out of my comfort zone that I wouldn't even be able to see it anymore.

CHAPTER 14
THE START OF SUSAN NIEBERGALL FITNESS ONLINE

I decided to take a big step and take Susan Niebergall Fitness (SNF) online.

I love training people in person. I love teaching and being able to help someone access a particular exercise. I love the interaction with clients. I truly love all of it, and my in person business was growing wonderfully.

The downside was that I was starting to see the inherent limitations with in-person training. The amount of people I could actually help was limited, and between the prep time for each client and the actual training time (and/or commuting time), I wasn't helping nearly the amount of people I wanted to help. I wanted to find a way to be able to help more people on a larger scale. I wanted to reach more middle-aged women and let them know that they can do this, and that it is not too late.

The answer was to coach online.

When I was looking for an online coach myself, at the time, I didn't quite understand it. My first thought was that online coaching was done through a Skype session, or something like that—and when people ask me about how online coaching works, that's what many believe. But if you think about it, a Skype session is just another type of in-person session, with regards to the time involved on the trainer's part. Once I started looking at online coaches and finally started working with Jordan, I saw how online coaching could work and how it could be the vessel to extend my reach and be able to help more people.

There seemed to be an extremely large number of online coaches already, and my first thought was: is there room for me? I had many long conversations with Jordan about this. He was blazing a trail in the online space, and told me that not only was there plenty of room for me in this space, but there was no one else like me in the space.

I hadn't thought of it in quite that way, but I knew I wanted to blaze a trail myself—especially for the middle age group. I wanted to be the example, the proof that an ordinary person can lose fat and build some muscle in her fifties and beyond.

A coach who has completely transformed her body and mindset in her fifties would likely pique the curiosity of similarly aged people. I just needed to find those people in the online space—wherever they may be.

As I began in the online space, I was overwhelmed and more intimidated than I can even begin to say. I was a retired educator, band director, and school counselor. My online experience was relegated to email and a minimal Facebook account. Instagram was brand new to me, as was YouTube and Twitter. I felt like a newborn, a newborn in her fifties. I had just retired from the school system and I was literally starting over. To say that I was overwhelmed would be the understatement of the year.

Starting a whole new business from scratch at my age is not an easy task, and moving all of the in-person business over to the online space created a bunch of new challenges. Learning the ins and outs of various social media platforms was the biggest mountain to climb. I had to learn things like the fine art of "hashtagging" a post so people can actually find you, how to format posts so they are easy to read (my Notes App has been my savior), how to film and format videos so they look clear, how to create headers, Instagram's famous Algorithm...I could go on and on.

Hearing my online colleagues talk about something called the Instagram algorithm was intimidating because I really didn't understand what it was, but my colleagues seemed to think it was really important.

It was all so confusing to me that it made my head explode.

To this day, every time I hear the word "algorithm," I put my fingers in my ears, and start saying "La-la-la-la." I made the conscious decision to forget the algorithm and keep focusing on my goal without it. Will my social media account grow more slowly as a result? Maybe. But that's OK.

At the beginning, I felt like I had to keep up with other fitness professionals who knew this stuff way better than I did. I didn't want to get left behind. There were times where it would create anxiety. Comparing yourself to others is never a great thing, and there were times I fell into that trap. But as time went on, I realized I couldn't compare my Chapter 1 to someone else's Chapter 12. I was at a different place, but I was learning quickly.

I was going to go at my pace.

As I am writing this, I am thinking, Wow, I've learned A LOT over the past several years. This old dog can learn new tricks, and the learning never stops. I have learned so much about training effectively, nutrition, and how the concept of nutrition for fat loss is not complicated at all. It may not be easy to execute all of the time, but it's certainly not complicated. The amount I have learned about social media is astronomical in my mind. It's not intuitive to me in the slightest, yet I am still able to learn and grow. Learning doesn't have to stop when you reach a certain age. It's a lifelong thing, as I was finding out then and continue to find out to this day.

The online fitness space was clearly dominated by people much younger than me—by twenty or thirty years, in most cases. This was another source of intimidation. All those young kids were working in an online space in which they comfortably grew up, posting multiple times a day with relative ease. I started the comparison game right away, which is probably the biggest mistake I could have made. I was trying to compare myself to someone who could be my own kid (I'm pretty much old enough to be everyone's Mom), and who were technology wiz kids compared to me. I felt like I wouldn't be able to keep up with them, and started wondering why anyone would listen to me with all of these younger fitness pros out there. They all looked great and had great-looking content. I was intimidated.

However, I also knew the online space needed older representation. I wanted to be one of those people, lead the way, and show middle-aged people that they can in fact, lose weight, feel better, and move better, regardless of their age.

I had to really get a hold of the comparison game. You know the quote, "Comparison is the thief of joy?" Well, there's a lot of truth in that statement. I didn't want my younger colleagues in the industry thinking less of me because I didn't know how to do much with technology, but I also didn't want to miss out on helping people through social media platforms that were foreign to me.

So, I had a choice to make (and this is really important and can be applied to a lot of things in life): I could say it was all too much for me at this stage of my life, succumb to all the intimidation and comparison, not dive into the online training world, and not reach my goal of helping as many people as possible,

OR I could dive in, learn, and do it anyway.

I chose the latter.

I had no idea how to even start, but I remembered one thing Jordan told me early on, when we were talking about me getting into the online space: Just Start. Start posting content online that will help someone.

It was that simple.

Jordan helped me understand that if I just focus on helping people, I would build trust with them over time. Then the rest (money, opportunities, etc.) will eventually take care of itself.

Helping people has and always will be my goal.

To quote Dan John, I want to "keep the goal the goal."

This is the exact same advice I give to anyone who asks me how to get back into their nutrition plan or their workout routine after being away for a while. You just start. There is no motivational song, quote, meme, or magic dust that will make that first step easy. You just have to grit down and do it. The best part is that you will never regret taking it. Ever. And the steps you take after that? They start to become easier. Less intimidating. Maybe even more fun, but it all begins with taking the initial step.

Sometimes, when you try to restart, it can feel overwhelming. There are so many things you want to get going again that it can become paralyzing, and you can stay stuck.

Instead of trying to get back to the gym three or four days a week for an hour-long workout, how about restarting by just walking every day? Start with that. Once that becomes a rhythm, then you can add to it. Breaking it down into less overwhelming chunks can be a great strategy for getting back to your routine.

So, I decided to take my own advice, grit down, and do this social media thing.

Trying to create a presence online wasn't going to happen overnight, so I knew I was in it for the long haul. Rome wasn't built in a day, so my online presence wasn't going to be, either.

When I first started posting content online, it was sloppy and probably not as organized as it could have been, but it was up there. Creating content did not come naturally at first, because I instantly became the Queen of Overthinking. I was trying to recreate a new wheel with each and every post. I was trying to find new and innovative topics and points of view to post every day.

The Perfectionist in me was alive and well, and just like the perfectionist who tries to lose weight by eating very few calories and only eating a small vocabulary of "clean" food, I eventually (and as perfectionists always do) found that it was unsustainable. Being so perfect about my online presence was going to be unsustainable for the long haul.

I was way too concerned about what other fitness professionals would think of me. Would they think I was stupid? Would they not agree with what I was posting? I am a people-pleaser by nature, so the thought of someone not liking me or not liking what I was doing was very uncomfortable. I was too focused on them, and getting their approval, but I soon realized that they weren't the people I was trying to help.

I think we all want approval from people to some degree. To say you don't give a damn about what people think is being a bit disingenuous, but making the sole focus of gaining approval your priority isn't the correct path to take, either.

Over time, I let go of gaining approval from colleagues and turned my focus to the people who truly needed my help. Once I started to do that, I also started to gain some respect from colleagues and other acquaintances in the industry along the way. It kind of took care of itself. When you look at coaches online, you will see a difference between those who are posting content that answers questions and have a takeaway strategy that can be implemented immediately, versus some who don't offer much in the way of specific help and are always trying to sell you something. Now, there is absolutely nothing wrong with trying to sell something, but when that becomes more of what you get over practical help, it may be a red flag. That person may not be in it to help you as much as they are to make some money.

For me, it was about keeping the goal the goal.

One big thing to remember about anyone on social media is that what you see is usually just a highlight reel. You will see their very best photos, or videos. You usually don't get a lot of behind-the-scenes type of stuff. One comment I get often is that people feel like I am relatable because I don't just post highlight reels. I do talk about when I am struggling, and how I deal with it. I want everyone to know I am not perfect. I am human. Sometimes, just knowing that others feel the same way as you do and have had similar struggles as you have had can be a game changer.

There are definitely people in the social media world who don't like what I post, and sometimes they will appear in my comments and quickly resort to third-grade name calling tactics. In the early days, that temporarily destroyed me. I could feel my blood boiling and my anxiety level rise, and I would worry about it incessantly.

But now, I take it as it comes. Those name-callers are obviously really unhappy people. Many do nothing all day except troll social media accounts and harass people. This phenomenon was eye opening to me when I first started, but now I see it for what it is.

I was also trying to find "my voice" in this online space. There are a gazillion online coaches who were posting about being in a calorie deficit, the importance of protein, and the importance of strength training, which are the cornerstones for fat loss. These were key points that I wanted to help people understand not only from a science point of view, but also from my own experiences. There was no one talking about these things in my voice, but my voice wasn't going to come through without consistent practice at writing and communicating. So, I gave myself a goal of posting on social media two times a day

At first, it was just a quote to get people thinking. Sometimes it was a video demo of an exercise, and oftentimes it was just regurgitating facts.

With my teaching and counseling background, teaching proper lifting technique and communicating with people was something I felt comfortable with and was good at. Giving a demo on how to properly perform a goblet squat or a DB row was something I loved doing. The learning curve of filming and being on camera was substantial, but like I have said over and over, you get better at anything with consistent practice. I sometimes look at my early videos and cringe, but it also reinforces just how far I have come over the years.

If I'm being really honest here, the amount of times I wanted to quit were numerous. But I didn't. I kept trying. And you know what happened? I got better. I learned. I became a little more proficient, every day.

Building a business is an interesting parallel to weight loss. So often I hear someone tell me they want to quit because they feel like it isn't working. They feel like they have been perfect with their nutrition and training and they don't see any progress—or, even worse, the scale may have spiked up so they panic. They are discouraged and want to quit.

And some do. But I can guarantee you this: the time you feel like quitting is the time you need to push through and keep going, because once you're on the other side of the struggle, good things start to happen. People give up too early. They give up when the scale does one of its crazy spikes thinking it's fat, when it's really due to water retention. If they would just keep going, change is just around the corner. I think we all need to learn patience and perseverance with everything in life, but with fat loss in particular.

The good news here is that as I continued working on my business, I surrounded myself with colleagues who were more than happy to help me, every step of the way. I started by trying to figure out everything myself and would literally spend hours working on something that many people would take minutes to do. I spent so much time being upset and being afraid that if I did ask for help, people would think less of me.

Eventually, I did learn how to ask for help. And my friends all came through with flying colors, all the time, without exception—and they still do.

This could be a similar path to your weight loss, as well. Trying to do it alone, doing things you think are right but may not be, and continuously spinning your wheels is not helping you like you think it is. Losing weight is hard to do alone. Asking for help may not always be easy, but it could be the very best thing you could do for yourself.

I also eventually hired a business coach to help advise me, keep me focused on my goal, and keep me headed in the right direction. Super lucky for me, that business coach was also my own strength coach, Jordan Syatt. Once again, Jordan pushed me out of my comfort zone, gave me structure, gave me deadlines, and taught me more than I ever thought I would learn. And the most important thing that I have learned is that I am still learning. I'll never, never stop learning.

Connecting with people is what I love most. I truly love to problem solve with people and give them actionable advice on how they can finally start to see progress. So many have struggled the exact same way I struggled. I can feel their frustration, because I walked in those shoes for many, many miles. I understand completely.

Being a good listener is imperative in this job. Humans all want and need to be heard. I learned this early on in my school counseling days. I had numerous parents walk into my office extremely angry at a teacher, administrator, or even at their own child. They walk in the door and they put up a defensive wall. They are frustrated and angry. My goal as a counselor was to break through that wall and get them to talk openly about their concerns. When the parents walked in the door, my job was to listen, because once they felt like they were heard, the wall went down, and we could then proceed and solve the problem.

As my online coaching business grew, I soon found the one thing that was going to keep me from helping as many people as I could: time. With one to one coaching you are inherently limited with how many people you can help just like in-person coaching. Writing programs, monitoring progress, emails, phone calls, watching client videos, etc. for each client takes up a lot of time. With only so many hours in the day, the number of people I could help had a ceiling.

Jordan had taught me how to create systems for my online coaching so I could be as efficient as possible, but even with that, I was feeling the limitations. I didn't want to be limited in the way I could reach people and actually help people with their goals.

So, as Jordan and I got to know each other more and he saw how I was interacting as a member of his Inner Circle, he provided me the perfect opportunity to help keep my goal the goal.

Little did I know that back when I joined the Inner Circle, it would prove to be another life changing event for me.

I was about to join forces with Jordan in the Inner Circle where our mutual goal of changing the world by helping as many people as possible will be alive and well.

CHAPTER 15
THE INNER CIRCLE

Online communities are in abundance. You can find online communities on every platform, and in every corner of the internet. Some communities are based on common interests (fitness, cooking, music, etc.) while others may be related more to age (Fit Over 40), or education, hobbies, faith, humor...there is a group or community out there for basically everyone.

On Facebook, they are called Groups. You can search on Facebook and find a group for almost anything you can think of.

Online groups can provide a sense of belonging. They can connect you with like-minded people you can communicate and share your journey with, and they can make you feel like you are part of something.

When you are trying to lose weight, having a community where you can share your struggles and your wins can play a huge role in your success. Feeling like you aren't the only one struggling to stay within your calories can be a game changer, and it can really help you to keep moving forward towards your goals.

But none of the communities out there in the internet world are like the Inner Circle.

The Inner Circle is a paid membership online fitness community that was created by Jordan Syatt back in 2015. Not everyone can afford the price tag of one to one coaching, so Jordan wanted to find a way to provide help, guidance, and support at a more affordable price point, thus expanding his reach and being able to help more people as a result.

Every month, the Inner Circle provides workouts, nutrition guidelines, metabolic circuits, detailed videos on exercise technique, videos on mindset, and recipes. But the best part about the Inner Circle is the community of people themselves.

I became a member of the Inner Circle in its early days, and what I found were incredible, well-constructed workouts, easy-to-follow nutrition guidelines, great exercise technique videos, and something I have not seen any other online communities do: discussions and content surrounding mindset. Mindset is really the most important part of a fitness journey. How we think affects everything, whether it's how we think about food ("good" vs. "bad"), or how we view our own ability to succeed. Our mindset leads the way, and the Inner Circle was hitting it head on.

In addition to the monthly content, the Inner Circle also has a Members' Portal full of manuals, videos, workout programs, and other helpful resources, as well as a Facebook-based community where members can interact with each other. Members post questions, they post about their successes, they post about their struggles, they support and hold each other accountable, and they even post videos of themselves performing exercises so they can get some critique and helpful tips.

If you've never been a part of an online group or have never really looked into them, as you start looking at them, take special note of the vibe or culture of the group. Are questions being asked and answered? Are people's posts getting responses? Are the responses positive and supportive?

All of these components comprise the culture of a group, which is at the heart of the membership.

One thing I noticed right away was that the culture of the Inner Circle was unlike any group I had ever been in. The Inner Circle Facebook group was not my first rodeo. I had been in many groups, and most started off fairly positive and supportive—but ultimately, one of the moderators would have to hop in to remind everyone of "the rules," which usually centered around being positive, not tolerating put downs or name calling, etc. Invariably, those kinds of negative comments would crop up sooner or later. It happens in almost all groups.

But not this group.

The culture in this group was different from the beginning and, if I am being completely open here, a group culture bleeds down from the top. Jordan set the bar with his positivity and encouragement from Day One, and it trickled down from there. He set the example, and lived by it for all to learn and live by as well.

As a member, I became more involved in the community and naturally started encouraging others, answering questions, and supporting whomever needed a little push or words of encouragement. I became a "regular," one of those people who was in the group every day. I loved being in there, I loved the content, and I loved making new friends.

The Inner Circle was home.

As time went on, my involvement with the Inner Circle grew. Jordan and I had several conversations about me becoming more officially involved with the group. He wanted to bring me on board as a co-coach with him in this community. Becoming co-coaches in this group seemed like a perfect match. Our goals aligned, our values were exactly the same, and we felt like we could be better together.

On paper, the partnership of a fifty-eight-year-old woman and a twenty-seven-year-old man seemed borderline ridiculous. The age gap would be tremendous. You'd think we would have nothing in common, very different goals, and very different perspectives.

The reality? None of the above was true. In fact, we would go as far as to say, our partnership is not only the most unique in the industry, but as close to perfect as you could get. Our goals and our ethics are the same: we want to positively change the lives of as many people as we possibly can.

We both genuinely care. We both have senses of humor (although I am no match for Jordan in this category), we both have a childish streak in us (pretty equal here), and our backgrounds (his in human behavior and mine in teaching and counseling) both play a significant role in our ability and desire to help people.

We think the same way and have almost everything in common. Jordan and I have a running joke that we are always on the same page. We are very much alike—but one area in which we weren't alike was planning.

I am a planner. I came to this partnership from thirty-three years of being an educator. Planning plays a huge role in being a teacher and a counselor. I like to think things through, sketch out a plan, and follow it through. I like to know what's coming.

Jordan, on the other hand, is more of a go-with-the-flow kind of guy. He was not as much of a planner. He likes the freedom and creative potential of going with the flow. You might think this could be a potential area of conflict, but I think it has instead become an area of growth and strength for both of us.

Over our time working together, we have both headed toward middle ground. Jordan is a much better planner, and I have certainly learned to let go and go with the flow more.

Old dogs can learn new tricks.

So, the best and most unique partnership in the fitness industry was official.

Jordan and I set out with one goal: to change the world by helping as many people as we possibly can.

Every month, I hop a train up to New York from D.C. and I spend a few days working on the monthly Inner Circle Edition with Jordan.

Editions come out monthly, and contain:

- The workouts for the month

- The nutrition guidelines for the month

- In-depth exercise tutorial videos

- A video from us on some aspect of mindset for nutrition, training, or just life in general

- Short metabolic circuits

- Special downloadable manuals or guides

- Video courses

- Recipes

We spend a lot of time planning out each Edition, and then we film all the videos. We also record a podcast together, and do a Facebook Live Q&A with our community. We want the Inner Circle to continue to be the premier online fitness community in the industry by producing quality, helpful content at a price point that is affordable.

One of our biggest accomplishments with the Inner Circle to date was hosting our first annual Inner Circle Retreat in Austin, Texas. We had several speakers (including ourselves) who spoke on relevant topics to our membership, we had a group workout in the world famous Onnit Gym with opportunities for us to help our members with technique and give them feedback, and we had plenty of time to socialize and get to know each other even more. To say it was a success is an understatement.

What had become quickly apparent was how our online community had brought people together from all over the globe via the internet and how the relationships with each other had grown. When we all met in person, it felt like we were seeing old friends we hadn't seen in a long time.

The feeling of normalcy was outrageous. It was remarkable to witness.

That's what a great online community will do: cultivate relationships by providing a safe and supportive space in which members can share, support each other, applaud the wins, and hold each other accountable. Time and time again, it has been shown that feeling like you aren't alone or that you aren't the only one going through something can make the difference, not only in a fitness journey but in life.

We want to continue to grow this Retreat over the years and make it one of the premier events of its kind in the fitness industry.

Jordan and I want to continue to learn how to best utilize our respective strengths to better help our community and change the world in the process. We truly believe there is not another more dedicated and more powerful duo in the fitness industry.

We want the Inner Circle to continue to be the standard that all other groups look up to. We want to not only continue to provide high quality workouts, nutrition guidelines, videos, manuals and an entire Members Portal full of more content than any place on earth, but even more importantly, we want to cultivate the culture.

Ultimately, it's the culture that will bring on the change, not a specific workout or guideline. That's why we're different. That's why the Inner Circle is unlike any other place on the planet.

And I am beyond blessed to be a part of it.

The Inner Circle came into my life at just the right time for me, on a personal and professional level.

At this point in my life, I finally started to feel like I had figured things out. My nutrition was on a roll. I was maintaining a new weight, which I had never been able to do before. I was building strength and muscle, and my mindset overall had completely changed. I had never before felt at such peace with myself and with my body. To be my age and to be strong, and to feel the best I have ever felt in my life was truly life changing.

I started a business after retirement that grew more than I could have ever imagined. I took risks, made a ton of mistakes, got way out of my comfort zone, and am now a co-coach in the best online fitness community in the industry, alongside the brightest mind in fitness who has become part of my family.

I would say life is pretty damn good.

CHAPTER 16
HOW TO OPTIMIZE NUTRITION FOR FAT LOSS AND MUSCLE BUILDING

One thing I have learned over time is that the concept of losing fat is simple: eat fewer calories than your body needs and be in an energy deficit, and you will lose fat. The concept is simple.

But if it's so simple, why do so many people struggle with it?

It's simple, but it's not easy. There is a big difference.

I am all about keeping things as simple as possible, and that includes losing fat, so let's dive in and talk about why people struggle to lose fat, and what you can do to lose fat slowly and sustainably.

One big reason people struggle with fat loss is that they make their workouts the priority, instead of their nutrition.

Think of fat loss this way:

Fat loss is a car, with a driver and a passenger. The driver of the Fat Loss Car is nutrition. Without the driver, you will go nowhere. Working out is the passenger. Workouts can be a great navigator and help you get to where you want to go, but they are not the driver.

It is interesting when people reach out to me completely frustrated because they aren't losing fat, and all they talk about is their workouts. How many days a week they workout, how they have added two additional classes per week, how they are going to add running to the mix. They think they aren't doing the right type of exercising, they think they need to add more cardio, they think they need to add more strength training.

It has to be the workouts. It has to be the passenger in the Fat Loss Car, right?

Wrong.

I never hear any mention whatsoever about nutrition. No mention of the actual driver of the Fat Loss Car. No mention of how many calories they are taking in, no mention of how much protein they are eating. Nothing. It's all about workouts.

I think we have found the problem.

Workouts are the easy thing to fix. Adding another class, adding more cardio, adding another round of High Intensity Interval Training, that's easy. What's not as easy (or as fun) is fixing your nutrition.

Many people think their Fat Loss Car is being driven by their workouts, when it's actually driven by nutrition. Nutrition will always be the priority for fat loss. Let me repeat that one more time: nutrition will always be the priority. If you are not in a calorie deficit, you will not lose fat. Again, we're back to simplicity.

Some other reasons why people struggle with fat loss:

- Thinking "eating clean" is all you have you have to do. While eating clean is great from a nutrient perspective, foods that you consider clean also have calories. Sometimes, they have a lot of calories. All calories count when you are trying to lose fat, and often we lose sight of healthy calories.

- You eat "intuitively" before you have learned about calories, portion sizes, and protein grams. Eating intuitively is an advanced skill that is learned through practice of counting calories and learning portion sizes. When you learned to ride a bike, most likely you started on a tricycle, got good with that, and progressed to a two wheeler with training wheels, got good with that, then on to a regular bike. You weren't given a two-wheeler and off you went. You had to learn, and progressively work your way to a bike without training wheels. Nutrition is the same way. Jumping from the beginning (never having counted or tracked calories before) to the end (intuitively eating) usually ends up in frustration and spinning your wheels. You will benefit greatly from the education you receive from putting in the work: tracking your calories, weighing and measuring your food, and logging it every day so you have a visual on your consistency. All of this sets you up for a life without having to track, if you don't want to.

- Thinking hunger is an emergency. We all can fall into this trap when we experience those initial hunger pangs where our stomach starts to growl. Our impulse is to go grab something to eat to take care of the hunger. We automatically grab something at the first sign of hunger because we don't want to be uncomfortable, but there is a big difference between being uncomfortable and starving. When you are trying to lose fat, you shouldn't be starving, but you should experience hunger—and experiencing hunger is not an emergency. I used to be the queen of always having a protein bar in my purse when I was out and about, "just in case." Just in case of what? I was going to be out and about running errands, not lost in the wilderness for two days. Learning to be comfortable with being a bit uncomfortable is a necessary part of losing fat. We don't need to respond with food every time our stomach growls. Sit with it, experience it, and you will find that initial hunger will dissipate and you will be just fine.

So let's keep the simple theme going and talk about how you can set yourself up for fat loss success with your nutrition. First, we have to understand a few things before we dive in:

- It does take work.
- It does take time.
- It does take consistency. Not perfection, but consistency

The key to losing fat and keeping it off is finding a way of eating that is sustainable and practical for your life. So, what diet is best for you?

Is it Keto?
Is it Paleo?
Is it Flexible Dieting?

The great news here is that they all work. Yep, every single diet or way of eating will work for fat loss, if—and this is a big IF—you are in a calorie deficit. Eating fewer calories than your body needs. It all comes back to that.

That's the great news. Before choosing a diet with my clients, I like to have people ask themselves a very important question (and I want you to do the same right now):

Can I see myself eating this way for the rest of my life?

If the answer is yes, then you have found a way of eating that will work for you! Keep going with it!

If the answer is no, then why would you do it? Why spend time with a diet that doesn't allow you to eat the way you want? Why spend time with a diet that you won't be able to stick with, and that will keep you spinning your wheels over time?

It makes more sense to find a way of eating that you love, that allows you to include any and all foods in your diet that you want, and that allows you to maintain that way of eating forever.

Keeping It Simple

Many people will tell you in order to lose fat, you need to precisely calculate every single macronutrient. While that is certainly an option, (and maybe even a good option, if you are a professional athlete or competitor), it is definitely not necessary if all you want to do is lose fat.

The two priorities for nutrition when it comes to fat loss are:

Overall daily calories (eating in a calorie deficit)
Overall daily protein

How to Create a Calorie Deficit

There are many formulas out there for creating a calorie deficit, and none of them are a slam dunk guarantee. They are all just starting off points. Finding a calorie deficit for you will require trial and error. So let's start here:

Take your **goal weight (in pounds)** and multiply by 11, and then multiply your goal weight by 12.

Note: Goal weight is what you think you might *want* to weigh. You don't ever have to weigh that amount. Think of it as a weight you feel you are at your leanest. If you like how you feel and how you look prior to reaching that weight, then great! You're done. The primary purpose of picking a goal weight is to use it in this calculation.

For example: Goal weight is 150 pounds.
150 x 11 = 1650
150 x 12 = 1800

Your calorie deficit starting off point would be between 1650-1800 calories per day.

Why a calorie range, and not a single number?

The chances of you hitting an exact number every single day is slim to none, and it is not the most flexible approach.

Missing a target day-in and day-out can start to play with your mindset. You can start to feel like you are failing, which can lead to a negative way of thinking such as: Screw it, what's the point? I am just not able to lose fat

Instead, have a calorie range which will allow you way more flexibility and give you a much better shot at hitting your target range. It is way more flexible, and way more doable.

So, based on a goal weight of 150 pounds, your daily calorie range is 1650-1800

Staying at towards the top end of the range will be a little more sustainable, but falling into the range would be the goal.

Now that we have that taken care of, let's move on to the Silver Bullet of Fat Loss: Protein

PROTEIN
The benefits of protein in your diet are numerous, but for the sake of simplicity, let's talk about the three most important benefits of protein from a fat loss and aging perspective.

1. Of all of the macronutrients, protein will keep you feeling fuller for a longer amount of time. While trying to lose fat and being in a calorie deficit, this is huge.
2. Protein has the highest thermic effect of all of the macronutrients. In simple terms, this just means that your body has to work harder to digest protein than other macronutrients, which means more calories burned. Huge win for fat loss.
3. Protein is the only macronutrient that will assist in building lean muscle mass. The more muscle you have, the more calories you will burn.

And here's the kicker (super important): as we age, we lose muscle mass. This starts at around age thirty, to the tune of five to seven pounds of muscle mass lost per decade. While we lose fat, we do not want to be losing muscle mass as well. Mother Nature is already trying to do that on her own.

While that sounds almost like a death sentence, the reality is it's all preventable, and reversible. We can not only maintain our muscle, but we can also continue to build muscle. Adequate protein is crucial.

How Much Protein Should I Eat?

Let's keep this simple too.

Goal Body Weight (in pounds) x 1 = protein grams per day

For example: Goal Body Weight = 150 lbs.

150 x 1 = 150 grams of protein per day

This is the number to aim for. Will you hit it every day?

No, probably not, and that's OK. You won't ruin anything.

Just aim for it.

Does this seem like a lot of protein? It might, if you are new to tracking protein, and it may seem impossible to get that much protein, but I can tell you it's easier than you might think. Here are a couple of quick tips to increase your protein:

Create a protein "cheat sheet" that includes:

- All of the protein sources you love
- A variety of portion sizes
- Calories for each
- Protein grams for each

Add to your list as you go along. This will become your go-to sheet for everything protein, and will make meal planning much easier.

If you are looking to increase the amount of protein you are consuming, look to increase the portion sizes of the protein sources you already eat. Instead of four ounces of chicken, make it five. Instead of a a half cup of greek yogurt, make it a full cup. That adds up quickly.

Before you know it, you will become a protein expert and will easily be hitting your protein goals.

Wait, What About Carbs and Fats?

Staying with our "keeping it simple" theme, let's briefly touch on carbs and fats.

Do You Have To Track Carbs and Fats in Order to Lose Fat?

The short answer? No.

The most important factor in fat loss is being in a calorie deficit. Eat fewer calories than your body needs, and you will lose fat. It doesn't matter where those calories are coming from; as long as you eat in a deficit, you will lose fat.

Here's an example: If you eat nothing but Twinkies, you can still lose weight if you are in a calorie deficit. But make no mistake here: you will feel terrible. Twinkies don't have any nutrients in them, you will be hungry all the time, you aren't going to feel well, and it's definitely not in the best interest of your health to take this for a test drive. Regardless, you will lose weight.

The point here is that a calorie deficit is king. It's always best to eat mostly nutrient-dense foods that will fill you up—and include an occasional Twinkie along the way.

The second most important factor in fat loss is protein, for all the reasons explained above.

Whatever calories you have remaining in your goal range after including your protein can come from carbs or fats, based on your preference.

Can you track carbs and fats? Of course you can, but it is not necessary for fat loss. Keeping your calories in check and aiming for your protein goal is what matters the most.

Tracking Your Calories and Protein

Tracking calories and protein is one of those things that sounds awful and tedious to do, but the reality is with all of the cool apps on the market these days, it has become easier and easier to do.

Apps are great to use as a food log, a place to conveniently keep track of what and how much you are eating.

Some of the more popular apps I have seen people use are:

- My Fitness Pal
- Lose IT
- Mike's Macros

There are a bunch more as well. But you don't even have to use an app to track. I never did (and still don't). As I mentioned before, I track on a simple spreadsheet I created myself, and I use Google and the FDA website to find out calorie counts and protein grams per serving. For me, this works great, but there is no real right or wrong way to do this. You need to find what works best for you, and that may mean trying a few different options until you settle on one that works.

I recommend everyone to go through a period of tracking calories and protein, as well as weighing your food, for a period of time. It's the main way you will learn portion sizes, which is where so many go wrong. Most people don't have horrific diets; they just eat too much. They think they are eating four ounces of chicken, but they are really eating six ounces. Those extra two ounces add up, and can result in major miscalculations when we are trying to count calories and protein.

Without experience, human beings stink at estimating portions and calorie content. The way to get better at that is to practice. Weigh your food. Track what you eat and drink. Tracking and weighing is not something you will have to do forever, but it's the best way to learn so that when you are ready to not track and weigh your food anymore, you will have gained so much knowledge that you become much better at estimating. When you can do that, maintaining, losing, and gaining become much easier. Put in the time and learn. It will pay dividends later

Can You Lose Fat And Build Muscle At the Same Time?

This is a question I get asked a lot, and the answer is: sort of.

You can't build muscle and lose fat in the same moment in time, because for one (lose fat) you need an energy deficit and for the other (building muscle), you need an energy surplus for optimal growth.

But you can, in fact, build some muscle while in a deficit and while in maintenance. The issue is it takes a long time this way. It's not efficient, and it can be super hard to accurately assess your progress, which can be extremely frustrating.

However, if you set up your program just right, you can do both with great success.

For example, let's say for three months you go into a fat loss phase. You dedicated three months to being in a calorie deficit consistently, tracking your calories and protein, and getting three to five strength workouts in a week.

After those three months, you slowly start to add calories back into your diet to get up to maintenance, and then even into a small surplus.

Now, let me stop right here for a second and calm the nerves. When people hear the word "surplus," they tend to think that means eating thousands and thousands of calories that will have you looking like a plump teddy bear. A surplus is not an uncontrolled eating frenzy. It is a controlled strategic way of increasing your calories to optimize muscle growth.

So, if you wanted to put on some muscle and go into a small surplus, what could it look like?

1. After coming out of your fat loss phase, try adding 300-500 calories over the course of a week, not by the day. Keep adding calories for one or two weeks or until your weight stabilizes.

2. You will have found your maintenance. I recommend hanging out there for a few weeks, just to get comfortable and to truly get to know what your maintenance is. Once you know your maintenance, you have so much power to do whatever you want, be it lose fat or put on muscle.

3. Then, add an additional 300-500 calories over the course of a week until you see weight gain of

about half a pound or a full pound per month.

Yes, the scale will go up, but if you do this as outlined above and hit the gym hard, the growth will be slow and controlled, and your muscles will grow which is the whole point. Make no mistake, you will put on some body fat. It's impossible not to, but that's OK.

At the end of six months, you will have done both: fat loss and muscle building.

I'll be talking a lot more in the future about building muscle. Be on the lookout.

How to Track your Progress

Most people use the scale as an indicator of progress, which is fine. The scale provides some great data, and it can be extremely valuable—If you understand how it works. It becomes a problem when you attach emotions to the number and then allow those emotions to drive what you do next.

The scale fluctuates every. Single. Day. Those daily fluctuations are mostly based around water. You're either holding onto water or letting go of water.

Comparing your weight from Monday to Tuesday doesn't mean much in the big picture. Consider the first thirty days of weigh-ins as nothing more than data collection.

After the first thirty days, start comparing numbers, but again not day to day. Compare your numbers month to month. When you start looking at the trends over time, you will see the real picture of what's really happening.

Think of it this way: when you invest in the stock market, you can check your stocks every day—but what happens with them day in and day out doesn't mean as much as what happens years from now when you want to cash them out. Most people are in the market for the long haul, not the quick fix. A stock could be down one day, and way up the next, but when it's down, you don't panic, and sell out. You stick with it. You keep going, because you are in it for the duration.

Same thing with your weight. It could spike one day, and then the next day take a big dip. You will drive yourself crazy trying to make sense of it all, so only compare your weight numbers month to month. You will be able to see overall trends and get a much better idea of how, exactly, your weight loss or muscle building is going.

I'd be remiss if I didn't mention other forms of progress that are equally as important (some may say more important) as scale weight:

How your clothes fit.
This is such an important indicator of progress. So often, your clothes will fit more loosely and you will feel better in them, but you will overlook it if the scale hasn't moved. The thing is, if your clothes are looser, you are LOSING FAT! Whatever you are doing is working! The scale hasn't caught up, but you are indeed losing fat.

Your measurements are changing.
Taking measurements regularly is super important. When your measurements change, it means you are losing fat. What you are doing is working.

Other signs of progress:

- You are lifting more weight in the gym.
- You are sleeping better.
- You have been consistent with your nutrition and workouts.
- You were able to go out to dinner and not feel guilty about what you ate.

There are signs of progress everywhere that aren't related to the scale. Make sure you recognize them all.

STRENGTH TRAINING

As you lose fat, you can also lose muscle if you're not careful, so while trying to lose fat, keep in mind that your primary goal is to maintain (or even slightly build) your muscle mass.

When we start losing muscle around the age of thirty, it becomes even more important to maintain muscle mass. To do this, you need to do two things:

- Make sure you're getting adequate protein (as we talked about before).

- Lift weights.

And when I say "lift weights," I mean heavy weights.

Not the tiny, brightly colored little hand weights you see in magazines, but utilizing DB's, barbells, cables, etc., and lifting as much weight as you can. An added benefit of lifting heavy weights is it helps improve and even increase our bone density, which can be a game changer as we get older. But again, I'm talking about heavy weights. As much weight as you can lift safely, with great technique.

One of the most common concerns I get about lifting heavy weights is, "But I don't want to get too bulky."

There's a couple of reasons why you don't have to worry about getting too bulky:

1. Testosterone. Testosterone is the hormone that leads the way for muscle gain. Men have a lot more than women do. A lot. Honestly, it's even hard for men to bulk up even though they have the testosterone. If it's hard for them, it's nearly impossible for women.

2. For optimal muscle gain, you should be in a calorie surplus — eating more calories than your body needs. That's how you "bulk up." Any women you have seen that have "bulked up" are eating in a very large surplus. Not a small, manageable surplus, but one in which they are eating way more calories than their body needs. And for many of them, that is purposeful based on their strength goals. So, if you are losing fat, (you're in a calorie deficit) and lifting heavy weight, it will be impossible for you to "bulk up" because you aren't eating enough.

While you are losing fat and lifting heavy weights, you will be building strength, maintaining muscle, and you very well may build a little muscle too, along the way. Lo and behold, you start to see that lean, toned, defined look you have been after!

And let's be crystal clear here. When you hear "lift heavy weight," no one is telling you to go to the gym and pick up the biggest DB you can hold and start squatting, lunging, and pressing it over your head.

What I am saying is that the word "heavy" is relative to the individual, and you should start wherever you are. But progressing in weight over time is necessary. Our bodies need continued resistance in order to maintain and build muscle and to improve and increase our bone density. Not to mention, the confidence you will get as you progressively get stronger and can lift heavier weight is something that will carry over into all aspects of your life.

A couple of weightlifting tips

1. Try to lift two to four times a week.

2. If you are completing all your repetitions fairly easily, you are ready to increase the weight used.

3. Weightlifting is not supposed to be easy. It is supposed to challenge you and take you out of your comfort zone. But that's OK. As a matter of fact, it's necessary.

4. Like anything else, consistency is key.

A sample Weight Training Week could look like this:

	MON	TUE	WED	THU	FRI	SAT	SUN
2 Days A Week	Total Body			Total Body			
3 Days A Week	Lower Body		Upper Body		Full Body		
4 Days A Week	Lower Body		Upper Body		Lower Body		Upper Body
5 Days A Week	Lower Body	Upper Body		Lower Body	Upper Body	Accessory Conditioning	

*Accessory / conditioning: Accessory exercises generally focus on one specific body part and are used to improve bigger lifts like squats, bench press,, etc. Conditioning can take the form of High Intensity Interval Training (IIIIT), short metabolic circuits (short duration circuits with weights), or any other form of cardio you like.

**Full body workouts includes upper body, lower body, and core exercises.

What About Cardio?

Cardio is extremely beneficial for heart health as well as mental health, but contrary to what you might think, cardio is not necessary for fat loss. Yes, that is right. Cardio is not necessary for fat loss. But that doesn't mean you should not do some cardio. In fact, adding some cardio to your exercise routine is a great idea. The benefits to your heart, your mind, and your overall health are massive.

So, as a reminder, what is necessary for fat loss?

But can cardio be helpful in the fat loss process? Absolutely. It can be, and it should be.

A couple of things to keep in mind:

- If you want to change your look, become leaner, more toned, and more defined, then strength training needs to be your priority.

- Adding cardio to your strength program can be extremely beneficial to your overall fat loss, and of course great for the heart and mind.

- Where most people go wrong is assuming that cardio is what will change the way they look by giving them lean and defined muscle, so they prioritize cardio over strength training.

Cardio could be simply walking (that's what I do), riding a bike, going for a run, or jumping rope. It doesn't have to be marathon sessions on the elliptical. I am a big proponent of moving in some way, shape, or form every single day. If you are not a fan of cardio, find something you like (or at least don't hate) and learn to incorporate it into your routine.

Just remember that from a fat loss perspective, strength training is the priority, with cardio getting the assist.

Mindset

The main principle of fat loss is simple:
eat less food than your body needs.

That's it. Stay in a calorie deficit, and you will lose fat. It's pretty simple, but regardless, so many people are struggling to lose fat. The reasons why can be pretty complicated and probably a topic for my next book, but in a nutshell, it's because of how we've been brought up to think about food. So many of us were brought up thinking some foods are "good" foods, and some are "bad" foods. With that mindset comes all sorts of unrealistic expectations that are surefire killers to any successful fat loss program.

"I can't eat a certain food because it will make me fat." This mindset is where we get ourselves into trouble. Not only is it not true, but it is no way to live. You can include any foods you love into your diet; you just need to account for them.

I love donuts. I regularly include donuts in my life, because, well, because they're donuts! Do I have them everyday? No. But when I do have them, I account for their calories in my overall daily calorie amount.

Nowadays, I hate the term "clean food." I used to use it all the time, thinking I was being smart, but the truth is that "clean food" means something different from person to person—and besides, it is not the end all, be all of weight loss. While the quality of food you eat is obviously important, especially from a health perspective, from a fat loss perspective, we're talking about quantity – eating less than your body needs. When you only eat "clean" foods and never allow yourself to have anything outside your severely restricted food bubble, things go wrong. It's not sustainable.

I used to think eating a donut or some pizza will cause me to get fat, and eating a salad will help me get skinny.

Look, food is just food. There are no morals attached to food. Some foods are more nutritious than others, yes, but there is a place for all kinds of foods in your diet, if you want to eat them.

Viewing foods as "good" versus "bad" just perpetuates an unhealthy relationship with food. It makes living and enjoying your life way more stressful and way more complicated than it needs to be.

I can remember going out to eat with my family and feeling full. Maybe even stuffed. I felt like I had gotten fat from that one meal. Panic and my irrational thinking started to kick in: "Uh oh, I have ruined everything. I gained fat. I shouldn't have eaten that." I felt horrible for allowing myself to get "so off track."

Side note here: these thoughts came after I had any normal meal at a restaurant, not an all-day fooding frenzy. One meal. And by most standards, it would have been considered "healthy."

I thought I had to "fix" it. I had to undo any of the damage I had done from going out to eat. So what did I do? I went downstairs and started doing crunches. I aimed for one hundred. My goal was to get rid of whatever fat I gained from the meal I just ate. I literally thought I could crunch it out. So downstairs I went, and I started crunching.

Is this sounding crazy yet? It makes no sense, logically, but when you allow your emotions to take over your decisions, logic goes out the window.

What I didn't understand was that the fullness in my stomach was a combination of:

- Stomach content (duh). Undigested food.

- A little bloating.

- A little water retention all over my body.

Logic should have told me that what was in my stomach was my meal as I had just eaten, and if I had really taken the time to think about it, I would have realized that I couldn't gain fat overnight. It just doesn't make sense.

So why was I allowing myself to go do something that made zero sense? Because I was allowing my emotions to take over. I allowed my emotions to dictate my actions.

This is something we've all done at one point in our lives. Whether it's regarding fitness, or our job, or our family, we've all fallen victim to allowing our emotions to take over and dictate what we do.

Take the scale for instance. Taking emotion out of the number on the scale is no easy task. Especially if you are in my age bracket and were basically brought up thinking if the scale goes up it's bad, and if it goes down it's good. Those emotions that you have held onto for so many years don't go away quickly. It will take consistent practice of weighing yourself, collecting the data, and objectively looking at it. It will also take a bunch of conversations with yourself where you keep telling yourself:

- I can't gain 2 pounds of fat overnight
- I can't lose 2 pounds of fat overnight

- I have more content in my stomach than usual, so of course I weigh more right now
- I ate more carbs than normal so I am retaining some water as a result
- Stop, you're being unreasonable (<--have said this to myself NUMEROUS times)

With nutrition, this can work like my example (doing something out of fear), or it can be on the opposite end of the spectrum. After you went out for that meal, you feel like you have screwed up, and you just say, "Screw it, might as well eat like any asshole the entire weekend, now." You proceed to turn one off-track meal into a weekend full of off-track meals, and then you start over on Monday once again. This is obviously not the right path, either.

How we think matters. What we tell ourselves matters, but *changing* how we think takes a lot of practice. Beliefs we have held for thirty or forty years don't go away with a flip of a switch; they take time to process, evolve, and change.

Keep after it. And the next time you start to panic because you ate one meal that took you over your calorie goals, try talking to yourself like you would a friend. You wouldn't tell your friend, "Oh shit, you've really screwed up. You've ruined it all." You would never in a million years tell your friend that. You would probably say something like, "Hey, it's OK. It's only one meal. You can't gain fat from one meal. Just hop back on track, and keep after it."

Try speaking to yourself that way. You deserve it.

CHAPTER 17
STRENGTH TRAINING WORKOUTS

Want to take a couple of strength training workouts for a test drive? I've got five workouts for you here that you can try.

The first and second workout require no equipment at all, but you can add weight if you want. And remember, if you are at home and thinking you don't have access to weights at your house, think again. Laundry detergent jugs, a box filled with books, and a backpack filled with books or even rocks are great weights you may have at your house. Think outside the box. We all have weights in our house; they just may not look like dumbbells.

The third, fourth, and fifth workouts require Dumbbells.

Give these a try! If you need help on the exercises listed, they are explained below:

Workout 1: Strength Builder

Instructions: Set the clock for 10 minutes and complete as many rounds as possible with perfect technique.

- Squats x 8

- Push Ups x 6 (you can elevate your hands, if you need to)

- Glute Bridges x 15

- Plank hold x 30 sec

Then do two rounds of:

- Squats x 12

- Close Grip Push ups x 12 (you can elevate your hands, just be sure to keep your elbows close to your side)

Workout 2: Now I Feel Ya

Instructions: Complete 5 rounds of the first circuit Rest 3 minutes. Then complete the second circuit as quickly as possible with great technique for 5 rounds

Circuit 1:

- Squats with pause down low x 10
- Reverse Lunges with pause down low x 10/leg
- Slow Bicycle Crunches x 10/side

Circuit 2:

- Push ups x 10 (Can elevate hands)
- Glute Bridges x 20

Workout 3: More Muscle Please

Instructions: Complete 6 rounds as quickly as possible with perfect technique.

- Dumbbell Romanian Deadlifts x 8

- Push Ups x 8 (can elevate your hands)

- Single Arm Dumbbell Rows x 10/arm

- Dumbbell Reverse Lunges x 8/leg

- Seated DB Overhead Press x 8

- Plank with slow reach x 6/side

Workout 4: Oh My Legs

Instructions: Complete 5 rounds of the first circuit, then complete 3 rounds of the second circuit. Rest at the bottom of each circuit as needed.

Circuit 1: 5 Rounds

- Bulgarian Split Squats x 6/leg
- Single Leg hip Thrust x 8/leg
- Lateral Lunge x 6/leg
- Slow Russian Twist x 6/side

Circuit 2: 3 Rounds

- Close Stance Goblet Squat x 10
- DB RDLs x 10

Workout 5: Big Shot

Instructions: Set the clock for 12 minutes and complete as many rounds of circuit 1 as possible with perfect technique. Rest for 2-4 minutes (whatever you need). Then set the clock for 10 minutes and complete as many rounds of circuit 2 as possible with perfect technique.

Circuit 1: 12 Minutes

- Goblet Squat x 8
- Push Ups x 8
- Single Leg Plank Hold x 20 sec.
- Single Leg RDL x 8/leg

Circuit 2: 10 Minutes

- DB RDLs x 8
- DB Bent Over Rows x 10
- DB Overhead Press x 8
- DB Bent Over Rear Delt Raises x 10

<u>BONUS WORKOUT: It's Ab Day</u>

Instructions: Complete Five rounds as quickly as possible. Your abs will love you!

- Plank with slow reach x 8/side

- Hollow Body Hold x 20 sec

- Plank Hold x 20 sec

- Slow Bicycle Crunch x 8/side

For more detailed instructions on these exercises, head over to Susan Niebergall Fitness on YouTube, where I have complete and detailed video instructions on all of these exercises—and many more!

Exercise Descriptions

Squat

Keep your feet about shoulder width apart, with your toes slightly pointed out. Sit your butt back and down at the same time, while keeping your chest up so someone standing in front of you can read the letters on your shirt. Keep your heels glued to the floor, and push your knees slightly out as you lower.

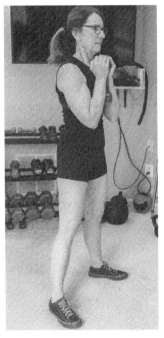
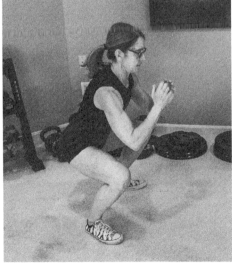

Push Ups

Brace your abs like someone is going to punch you in the gut. Squeeze your glutes hard. Send your shoulders back down to your back pocket (keep them away from your ears). When lowering into a push up, keep your elbows at 45 degrees to your body, not flared out to the side.

If you can't get a push up off of the floor yet, elevate your hands on a table, counter, or bench and practice the perfect push up position with full range of motion, and slowly lower the elevation over time.

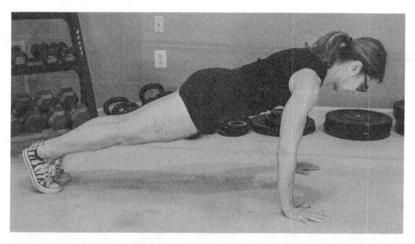

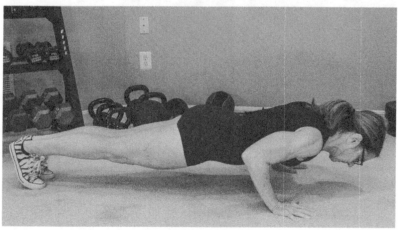

Glute Bridges

Lay on the floor with your knees bent and feet flat on the floor. Push down into your heels and raise your hips in the air.

Do a slight pelvic tilt at the top and squeeze the glutes! You can add a band around your knees for extra resistance.

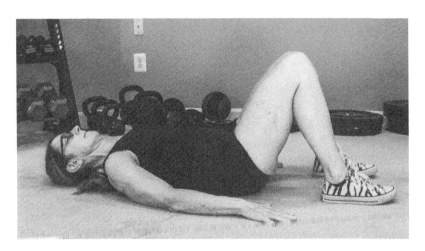

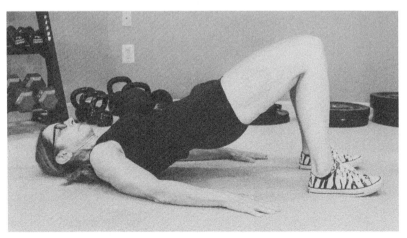

Plank Hold

On your elbows and toes, brace your abs like someone is going to punch you in the gut, squeeze your glutes hard, and send your shoulders down to your back pocket (shoulders away from your ears).

Keep all of this actively engaged as you hold your plank. Keep your hips level and try not to let your belly sag as you begin to feel it in your low back.

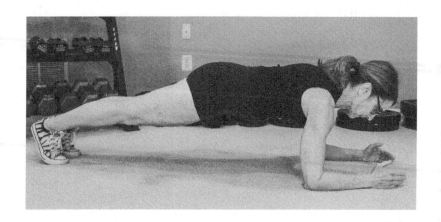

Close Grip Push Ups

Exact same technique as above, only keep your hands very close together—your thumbs should touch.

As you lower, elbows on this variation stay at your side. This is a tricep-focused movement.

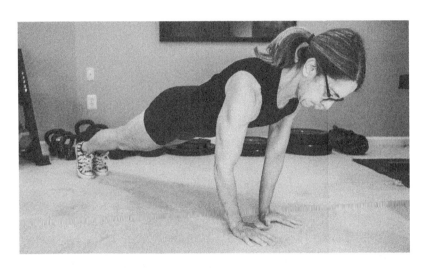

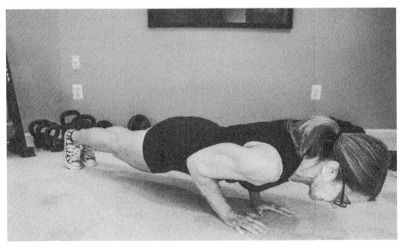

Dumbbell Romanian Deadlifts

Hold the Dumbbells on your legs as you send your butt back behind you, to try and touch the wall behind you. Keep your knees soft, and shoulders set back (don't slump).

This exercise is not about how low you can go; it is more about how far back can you get your butt. You should only be lowering to about your knees or just below.

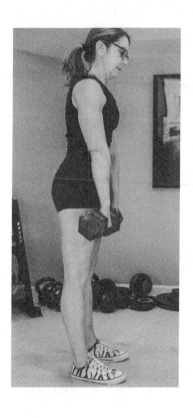
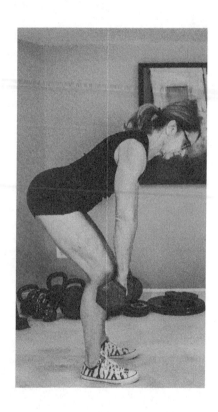

Single Arm DB Row

Get into a split stance with one hand on a chair or bench. Start with the arm long and row the DB back toward your hip until your arm is in line with your torso.

Don't over row and send your elbow high in the air like a lawn mower. Keep this controlled and squeeze the shoulder blade.

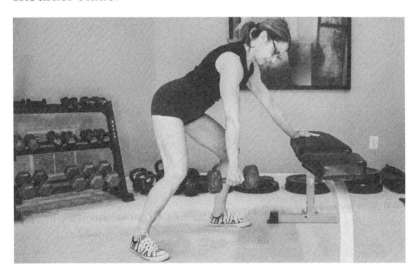

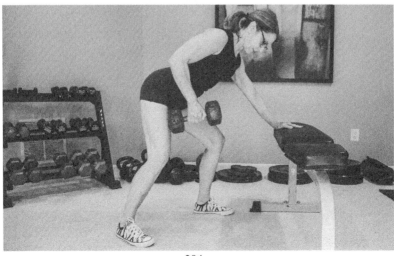

Dumbbell Reverse Lunge

Holding a Dumbbell in each hand, start with your feet together. Step back into a lunge position by bending both knees.

Weight should be on the front heel which needs to be planted into the ground the entire time, not on the back toes. Step back into standing. When in the lunge position, slightly lean forward to feel it more in your glutes.

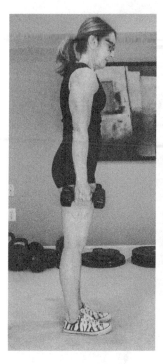
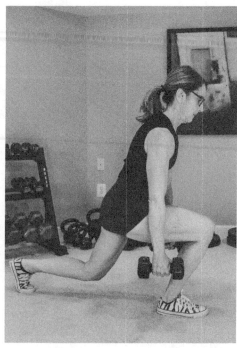

Seated Dumbbell Overhead Press

Hold Dumbbells just above the shoulders with palms facing each other. Press overhead aiming to get your biceps by your ears.

Be careful not to "shrug" your shoulders up. Lower the Dumbbells to just above the shoulders.

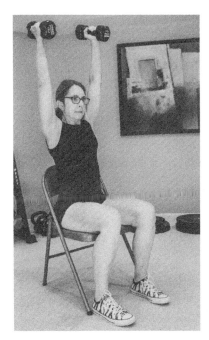
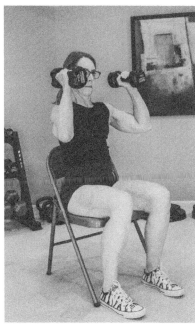

Plank with Reach

Get into a fully engaged plank (see Plank Hold description) and slowly move one arm so it reaches in front of you. Tap the floor without allowing your hips to rotate. This is an anti-rotation exercise, and is very challenging. You can try it from your knees first and progress to your elbows.

Brace everything super hard.

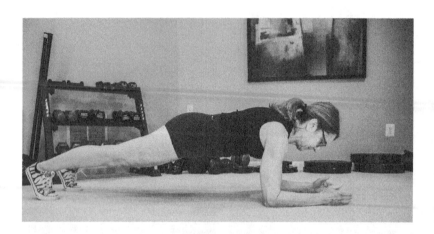

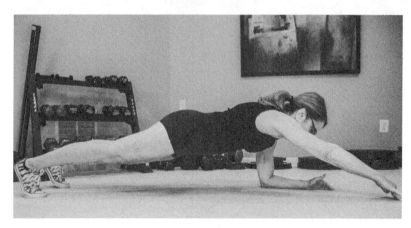

Hollow Body Hold

Lay on the floor with your legs straight and slightly off the floor, your arms overhead, chin tucked, and shoulders slightly off the floor.

Your body will make a banana shape. Keep pressing your back into the floor as you hold. If this is a little too challenging right now, put your arms at your side and raise your legs a little higher off the ground while pushing your back into the floor.

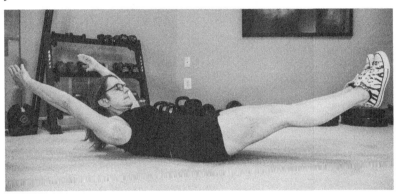

Slow Bicycle Crunch

Lay on your back with knees bent in the air at 90 degrees, hands behind your ears. Slowly extend one leg (keep the other knee at 90 degrees) and twist from the torso to the opposite side.

Your elbow should not lead the way. The torso leads the way. Slight pause at the twist, reset, and repeat on the other side.

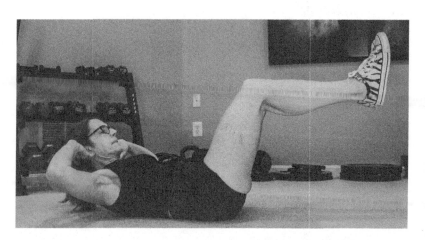

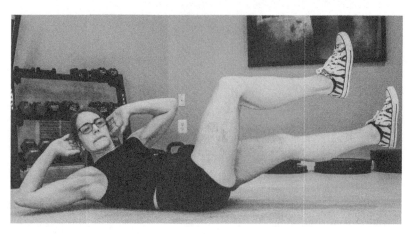

Bulgarian Split Squats

Elevate one leg behind you on a chair, box, or bench, preferably laces down. Make sure you have enough room to lower down without the front heel coming up off the floor.

Drive the back knee down, slightly lean forward and keep that front heel glued to the floor.

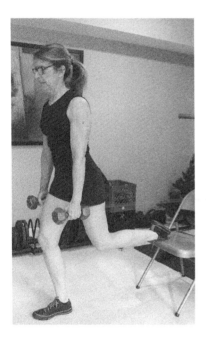

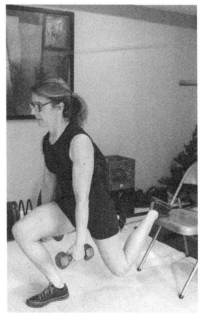

Single Leg Hip Thrust

Lay on a bench or other elevated surface so the edge of the bench is lined up with your armpits. Knees at 90 degrees. Lift one leg slightly off the ground, while keeping the knee bent.

Keeping your chin tucked, lower your hips and ribs, and push into the heel to get yourself back up in the hip extension position

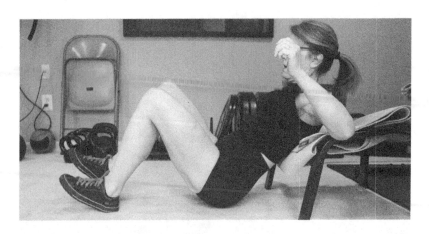

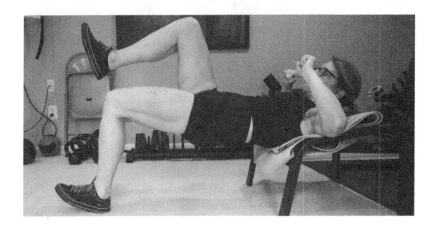

Slow Russian Twist

Sit nice and tall with a slight lean back, heels on the ground arms extended as an extension of your chest. They should point towards where the ceiling and wall meet. SLOWLY twist from the torso, not the arms. The arms have to stay in line with your chest (they will want to get ahead) and as you twist, you are still sitting tall and slightly leaned back.

For an extra challenge, lift your feet slightly off the floor and twist the same way, maintaining the position the entire way through.

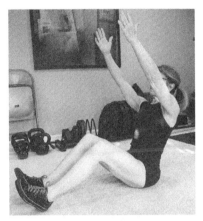
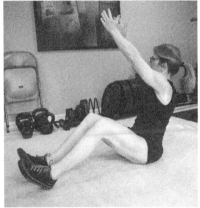
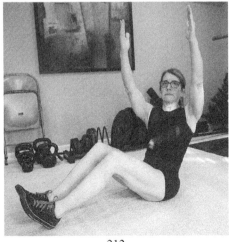

Lateral Lunge

Start with feet together, all toes pointed forward. Step out to the side, and sit your hip back (like you are going to sit down) while keeping your chest high.

One leg will be bent and the other should be straight. Push down into the heel of the bent leg to get back to the starting position

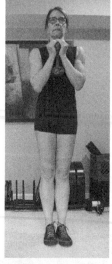

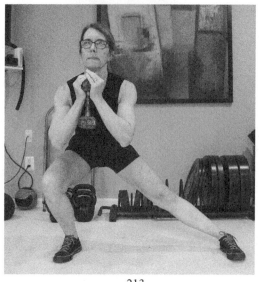

Close Stance Goblet Squat

Same as a goblet squat only your feet are together. This variation will be more quad dominant than hip dominant.

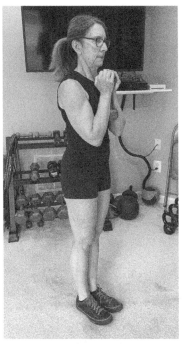

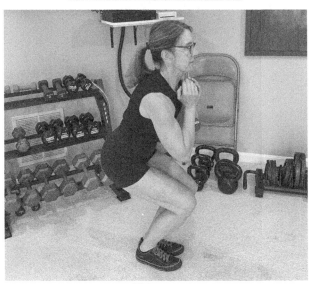

Single Leg Plank Hold

The exact same position as a regular engaged plank, just lift one foot slightly off the ground (Don't stick it way in the air).

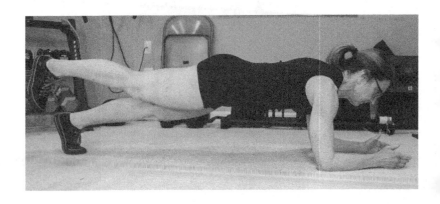

Single Leg RDL

Hinge at the hip and send one leg back behind you while you keep your chest high (don't collapse). Reach the back leg to the wall behind you. Standing leg has a soft knee. Hold the weight on the same side as the leg that is going back. Keep shoulders engaged and back.

*If balance is an issue, lightly hold on to something to help stabilize you. It will not take away from the exercise.

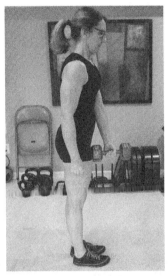

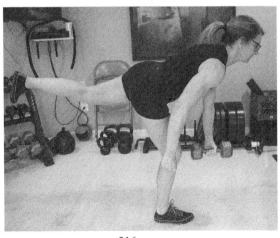

DB Bent Over Rows

Send your hips behind you (hinge). Your weight should be in your heels. Brace your abs. Chest will be slightly facing the floor. Row the DBs from the elbows back towards your hips. Be careful not to over row and send your elbows way up above your body

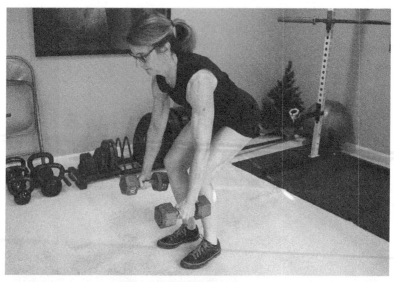

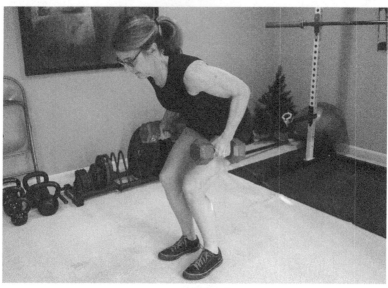

DB Bent Over Rear Delt Raises

Send your hips behind you (hinge). Your weight should be in your heels. Brace your abs. Pull the DBs straight out (not back), and squeeze the shoulder blades.

Keep the upper body still so you don't use momentum to drive the movement

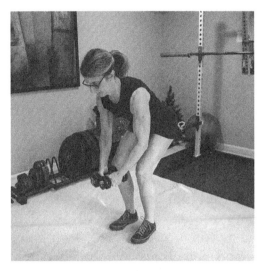

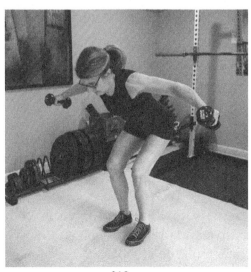

CHAPTER 18
IMPORTANT THINGS TO REMEMBER

As I close this out, I want to leave you with four final messages that I would love for you to keep in the forefront of your mind as you move forward. Trying to lose weight is not easy, and sometimes we get in our own way—especially with how we think and what we tell ourselves.

These messages can be game changers and can change your life forever. They did for me.

Get Rid of Timelines

How many times have you thought, "I should be losing weight faster," or even, "I should be lifting more weight by now." What do you think drives those comments?

This imaginary timeline you have in your head is a totally made up standard, and as a result, you get a case of what I call the Should Be's:

- I should be losing weight faster
- I should be lifting more weight
- I should be doing _____ diet
- I should be working out more

Any of these ever cross your mind? They've certainly crossed mine.

The Should Be's put unwarranted pressure on you to perform. They try to get you to believe there is some imaginary standard that you have to hold up to, or you are a failure.

But they're wrong

For some reason, you think when weight loss doesn't go as quickly as you want it to, there must be something wrong. You start thinking you need to make changes (drastic changes) because you aren't making progress. You aren't meeting the imaginary standard you have in your head, and pretty soon you find yourself restricting your calorie intake so much that you are miserable, can't sustain it for long, and you end up binging or massively overeating regularly. Then it's back to square one, yet again.

See the problem here?

This is a very common cycle that is often self-inflicted. You go through that cycle time and time again, all because you thought you weren't losing weight fast enough.

Fast enough for what?

Contrary to what we think, there is no finish line. There is no, "Aha! I've arrived!" moment. That only exists in our minds. The reality here is that you continue to evolve, grow, and change your whole life. It's never over. Well, until you're buried in the ground. I'd say it's over then.

This journey we are all on is for life, so stop putting pressure on yourself to "perform" at a certain pace. This isn't a race. There is no prize for finishing first. Once you can take the weight of unrealistic expectations off your shoulders, you will feel as liberated as you have ever felt in your life. For the very first time, you can actually enjoy the ride, all the ups and downs, accomplishments, failures, all of it.

After all, we only get one shot at this thing called life, right? We might as well enjoy every single second of it. Isn't that the point?

Let go of those timelines and enjoy the ride

You can't mess this up.

Seriously, you can't mess this up.

It doesn't matter how many times you got off track. It doesn't matter how many workouts you missed, how many diets you tried, or how many times you failed. As long as you get back on track, you will succeed.

That's a guarantee.

That's the beauty of this. Whether you have one off track meal, one off track day, one off track month, or even one off track year, as long as you hop back on track and keep going, you will succeed.

The road is not easy. It will not be quick. The concept of losing fat is simple: consume fewer calories than your body needs, but getting there takes time. It will try your patience like nothing else. You will want to quit multiple times as you swear it's not working, but if you just keep going, even when it seems insurmountable, your efforts and dedication will pay off, and you will indeed come out on the other side.

There is literally just one thing that separates those who are successful and those who are not: those that are successful stumble, but they get up, dust themselves off, and keep going.

That is the only difference.

You will make mistakes (as you have read, I have made a bucket load of them), you will have periods of time (could be months) that it seems like nothing is working for you. But that's OK.

Just keep going. Push through the resistance. Grit down.

Keep fighting, don't give up, and you will succeed.

Injuries

I talked a lot about the importance of rest days, and why they are critical for making progress with your workouts.

There can also be consequences from not taking adequate rest days not least of which are injuries.

I've had my fair share of injuries along the way:

- A shoulder impingement that required a shoulder scope–relatively minor procedure
- A full thickness rotator tear on the other side (as diagnosed by an MRI)
- A hip impingement
- Elbow tendonitis

The interesting thing to point out here is that through all of these injuries (over several years), I never missed a training day.

Not one.

And I say this to emphasize a couple of things:

1. You can literally train around anything
2. You can still make progress through any injury

The mental aspect of being injured is indeed the most difficult part. We get on a roll, we are seeing progress in the gym, and boom. Our shoulder is aggravated or our knee is irritated. Immediately, in our minds, we start thinking about how we have to take time off, and how we are going to lose all of our progress as a result We seem to lament on all the exercises we temporarily can't do. We get discouraged easily because things aren't the same, and often that leads to despair, and the whole "why bother" attitude.

I found a doc who specializes in movement and injury recovery. Dr. Matthew Clay and my coach, Jordan Syatt never once told me to stop working out. In fact, they both encouraged me to do just the opposite: Get in the gym and find what you CAN do.

That's exactly what I did.

I think taking complete rest may be a bit old school. Heck, knee replacement and hip replacement patients are up and walking the next day or even later the same day as their surgery. What I have learned is that when you keep moving, you allow blood flow to get to the injured area which helps to promote healing. The longer a joint stays sedentary, the longer your recovery will most likely take.

Now let's be clear, that doesn't mean pressing 100 pounds overhead with a shoulder injury.

It means, having common sense, being smart, and finding exercises you can do without causing pain.

Your workouts may look different, but that's ok. In fact it's great. You can still move and get strong with those exercises while your injury heals up.

And when you do that, you're keeping your head in the game. The worst part of being injured is the mental part, and the fear that goes with it. But once you get in there and find exercises you can do, you now have a new focus. Instead of focusing on all of the things you can't do, you are now focusing on what you CAN do and how you can get strong with those movements.

I learned very quickly that:

- Having an injury isn't the end. It doesn't mean it's over.
- Strength training is not inherently dangerous. Getting minor injuries (most are indeed minor) is

part of the game. And my doc often told me he would rather see me in his office because I was active, rather than seeing me because I was sitting around and being sedentary. The recovery is way different.

- Continuing to move and train in whatever way you can is the best remedy not only for the injury itself, but for your mindset as well.

It's Never Too Late

I want you to know, from the bottom of my heart, that it's truly Never Too Late to make whatever changes you want to make. Take it from someone who used to think it would never happen for her, who thought she was doing everything right and blamed everything for her lack of success except herself.

It's Never Too Late.

Look, I am no one special. I don't have "good genes" (unless you think obesity and heart disease are good genes, then I guess I hit the jackpot). I am not an athlete. I am about as uncoordinated as they come.

I am just an average person who struggled with weight for most of her life and couldn't get all the pieces of the puzzle put together until I was in my fifties, when I finally stepped up and took responsibility for what I was doing.

There were no shortcuts. No cleanses, no detox teas, and no overly restricting my calories. I did it the hard way—the right way.

It wasn't too late for me, and it's not too late for you.

The science of weight loss is the same for everyone. Finding a sustainable approach may look different from person to person, but here is your weight loss checklist, whether you are twenty, fifty, or eighty years of age:

1. A modest calorie deficit

2. Adequate protein intake

3. Strength training

4. Daily movement

5. Consistency

6. Patience

This is your weight loss recipe. It's not sexy, or even all that enticing, but it works for everyone, regardless of age.

Consistently follow it, and you, too, can change your life forever.

Listen, life is too short to be miserable on your diet.

Life is too short to keep beating yourself up for having a treat (please stop).

Life is too short to be afraid of attending social gatherings because you think you will ruin your progress.

Life is too short for super light weights—pick up the heavy stuff.

Life is too short to choose anything other than optimism.

It's never too late to do whatever you want to do.

That's probably the best gift that any of us have.

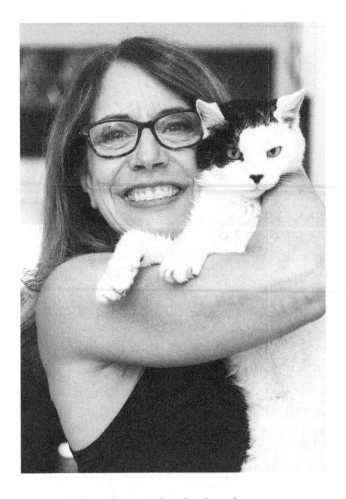

Thank you for being here.
Love You,
Susan

Where you can find me!

Please never hesitate to reach out if I can help you in any way. You can find me here:

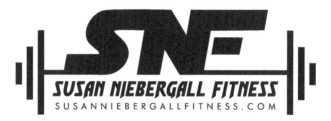

www.susanniebergallfitness.com - My website where you can learn more about me, nutrition, and training.

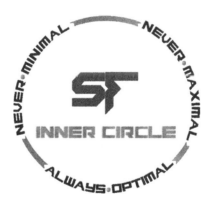

Syatt Fitness Inner Circle - sfinnercircle.com The premier online fitness community that I coach alongside Jordan Syatt, where we provide sustainable nutrition guidelines for fat loss, maintenance and muscle building, training programs for the gym or at home, video courses, downloadable manuals, and some of the most amazing recipes you will find. It is appropriate for anyone at any age and ability level, and includes the support of the most amazing community on the planet.

Instagram: @susanniebergallfitness I post content on nutrition, exercise technique, and info you can implement right away, as well as sharing my own training, current goals, and obstacles.

Facebook: Susan Niebergall Fitness Here I provide content that will help you every step of the way along your journey.

YouTube: Susan Niebergall Fitness I post tons of videos on nutrition, from tips to help you lose fat and when to take a diet break to nutrition strategies for building muscle at any age. I also have complete exercise tutorials and even some workouts you can try! Click **subscribe** so you will be notified when a new video is out.

Twitter: @ssniebergall1 (Susan Niebergall Fitness) Here you will find short, solid tips on nutrition and exercise.

Podcast: Strong and Lean at Any Age Podcast Here, I bring in leaders in the fitness industry and we talk about health, nutrition, and fitness at every age.

ACKNOWLEDGEMENTS

I have to give a huge shout out and massive hug to the following people who have helped me with this book project. This book would never have happened if it weren't for you:

Jordan Syatt, for changing my life.
Syatt Fitness, Syatt Fitness Inner Circle

Rico Incarnati, for taking the incredible shot for the book cover.
Enrico Incarnati Productions

Dan Weinel, for all of the amazing video and photo content.
Dan Weinel Visuals

Tina Leu, for the amazing photos.
Tina Leu Fotos

Deborah Haile, for helping me navigate this whole process.
Jonah Global Footprints

Judith Leishear, for making this book come to life!

earned so much from but most importantly is age is not an excuse for being fit. My blood essure is low enough to duce meds and I am wearing sizes smaller. It's a process nd with your inspiration, 'm in it for the long haul.

-Nancy, Encinitas, CA

helped me NOT GIVE A F@CK a the scale. Fluctuations - they happen! That on rest days, we rest (Like, actual.

-Katherine, Toronto, Car

What I learned from you is that 40 is not too late to pursue fitness goals. I am looking forward to breaking every paradigm that had bummed me out

-Maria, Guatemala

listened, you simplified and u reminded me of what I alrea ew and was afraid to put back o action.

n my hardest days, even wh ave every excuse in the wor

come back to that conversation and now where I need to be. Having you in my head and on my side is magical.

-Marie, CT

It's never too late to g strong! I really thought was over post 40, but y inspired me so much

-Safiyah, Lon

hat I have learned from you: ou have to keep your patience ants on and if you do, you can accomplish any of your goals, ter your age!

-Rose, Miami Fl

You can eat more food and still lose weight are in a calorie deficit. But don't add back t your exercise sessions.

-Sarah, S

om you I have learned the portance of having good m and knowing what to k for!

Age is just a number. It's never too late to get strong.

olis, M

at your age is not an excuse
not lift! Also, I've mastered
in ups thanks to you.

-Carla, Toronto Canada

our consistent and sir
messages and your
orgeous personality,
otivate me daily.

Karla, Melbourne, Austr

tting older doesn't mean
t I have to stop trying to
he healthiest I can be
ne.

-Jese, Sugar Land, TX

olutely love your co
body form. I have learned s
ch. You give me hope for h
my golden years.

-Victoria, San Die

He driver behind the fitne
goals is waaaay deeper th
looking good. The driver
literally I want to be heal
for a longer stretch of my

-Sara, I

Fit and Strong at any age is
possible! There's always
something new to le
row from.

ou
or
alia

Whyalla, South A

arned the proper form for a
h up from you.

You have taught me that MY prog
unique to me and takes many fo
more importantly, there is no d
is no rush, all I have to do is sh

Thank yo
-M